Circuit Training for Beginners

A 6 Week Beginner Home Workout Manual for Losing Weight, Gaining Energy, and Improving Self-Esteem.

By Andrew Hudson

are declared or implied. Readers acknowledge that the author is not engaging in the rendering of legal, financial, medical or professional advice. The content within this book has been derived from various sources. Please consult a licensed professional before attempting any techniques outlined in this book.

By reading this document, the reader agrees that under no circumstances is the author responsible for any losses, direct or indirect, which are incurred as a result of the use of the information contained within this document, including, but not limited to, — errors, omissions, or inaccuracies.

Table of Contents

Introduction

Many people across the world struggle with obesity or being overweight, and the problems that come with it are starting to become normal for a large chunk of the population. There are many possible reasons for why so many people are out of shape, the main ones being that unhealthy takeaways can be ordered just with a few clicks, having a healthy diet is portrayed as torture and most people don't know what it takes to lose weight.

The reasons above are just some of the reasons why 71.6% of the US population are overweight, that's almost three quarters! This means that most people in the US have thrown away their good health and now struggle with the consequence like, being more likely to develop fatal health-related issues, lack lots of energy by carrying around their excess weight and may be embarrassed by their own body.

If you feel as if you relate to any of the problems above or are worried about your health deteriorating, don't worry because this book will help you make the changes you need to escape the downsides of obesity or being overweight. I was once overweight and I know what it is like to experience some of the downsides that come with it, it was a tough time of my life and I thought breaking free from my unhealthy lifestyle was impossible. That's until I followed simple steps you can find in this book which began my weight loss journey.

I understand many people want to get out of their unhealthy lifestyle and lose weight to look better, feel more confident, or want to train for something like the army, or just lower the health risks. Whatever the reason is for you wanting to lose weight, I am here to support you along your journey.

My name is Andrew Hudson. I am a personal trainer who has recently taken a turn to writing because I know that I can help more people reach their fitness goals. I love helping people reach fitness goals for many reasons, mostly because I feel great when I see people manage to turn their life around for the good through fitness. That is also why I want to help you, although this isn't a 1 on 1 training session, you will still be able to progress towards your goal and feel great while doing so!

Circuit training is what this book is based on and it's a brilliant training method! This is because circuit training allows you can be exercise at home with little equipment, takes hardly any time to set up and is a quick workout that you can easily fit in a few times a week. Also, these circuits are quite fun if I do say so myself. This book will provide you with some great motivational tips, dietary advice, health & fitness information, weight loss tips and a wide range of exercises that will accelerate your weight loss progression.

The 6-week workout plan is what I hope for you to follow. This will gently ease you into a routine of exercise and a healthy lifestyle which will set you up for your healthy future. It doesn't end after 6 weeks because the information provided in this book will allow you to extend your routine further until you reach your fitness goal!

Exercising, learning, and breaking into a routine gets harder with age. That is why you should start now – you will not regret it! If you don't make this change now, then your health will only continue to decline, your body will not thank you for that in the future.

Your journey starts here, I wish you the best of luck and this book is your guide to your goals. Work at your own pace and follow the tips provided, I believe in you. If you are still sat on the fence, why not give this a go? You have nothing to lose...

Circuit Training for Weight Loss

This is the first book from the three-part series, "Circuit Training for Weight Loss". This series is for people that are looking to reach fitness goals at home with the training method: Circuit Training. Whether your goal is to lose weight to avoid health risks, to improve your health or if you are looking to lower your body fat percentage to look ripped/toned, then this series will help you out. Below you will find a brief description of each book and a summary of the series at the end, if you want to find out more, then search up the book titles to view the detailed description!

As this is the first book of this series, it is the most basic, but that doesn't mean that you won't be able to lose weight from it! This book is to get you into a simple exercise routine, will help you clean up your diet and give you an understanding of general health and fitness. This book is a great starting point to set you off on your weight loss journey, helping you break your old unhealthy habits so you can no longer fall under the obese or overweight category.

The second book of the series, "Intermediate Circuit Training", is the next step that increases the difficulty of the workouts, so you make quicker progress towards harder fitness goals. This still sticks with the theme of weight loss with circuit training and nutrition, but this book starts to branch out to slightly more advanced health & fitness information and starts to present motivational advice, so you stay on track with your fitness goal. This isn't for complete beginners, more for the average person looking to lose weight.

The final book, "High Intensity Circuit Training", is the most advanced book. The workouts in these books are shorter, but much more difficult because this book is to help people with difficult fitness goals. Goals like having a low body fat percentage and having a high lean muscle mass percentage are what can be reached by following this final book. This book also offers advice on how to adapt your mindset to reach challenging goals, information about how to boost your metabolic rate and many other ways to burn fat quickly to lower your body fat percentage while building lean muscle mass. This is for the more experienced fitness fanatics.

As you can see, each book from this series is like a steppingstone towards your final fitness goal. Each book goes up in difficulty and if you are looking to go from Fat to Fit, I highly recommend following each book 1 at a time to reach and maintain your goal of having your dream body!

Your Free Gift

The gift you'll receive is an eBook titled: The Circuit Training Weight Loss Bundle. This eBook contains many extras to help you lose weight at a quicker rate and be on top of your progress. In the beginner section of this book, you'll discover:

2 Extra Circuits that you can complete at home, these circuits are slightly more advanced than the ones provided in this book to encourage progression.

Secondly, you will find a checklist full of the optional equipment included in this book. Each piece of equipment has a link to where you can buy it a reasonable price. A list of all the optional equipment all linked. This will allow you to find the equipment for a reasonable price.

You will also find a food budget tracker - a spreadsheet that will allow you to keep track of how much you spend on food with the goal to help you save money in a healthy fashion.

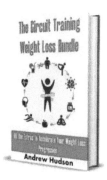

Follow this link for the free eBook:

https://hudsonandrew.activehosted.com/f/33

Join the Workout for Weight Loss Community

Living a healthy lifestyle is difficult, especially when you feel as if you are doing it all alone. That's why I suggest for you to join a community of others who are in your situation, this community "Workout for Weight Loss" will provide you with daily posts about weight loss and there will be many people that you can talk to, share experiences with and receive help from.

I aim to post twice a day, providing you with tips, tricks, motivation, workouts, diet plans and so much more to help you lose weight. Not to mention that I may host a few book giveaways every now and then. In a community, your chance of reaching your goals is much stronger and you may make many new friends in the process!

So, if you are looking for that extra help, please join my Free Facebook Group: https://www.facebook.com/groups/workoutforweightloss

Free "Circuit Training for Beginners" eBook

You may find that in this book there are a few links for you to follow which is inconvenient because you can follow a link through a paperback book without spending 10 minutes typing in 40-character links into your URL.

The links in this book are beneficial to help you progress further with your boxing ability and I don't want you to miss out on them. That is why I am giving you the free PDF eBook copy of this book so that you can access all the links with just a click.

To get the eBook, you will have to type in a short link into your URL (ironic I know...) and you will have the eBook emailed directly to your inbox.

So please type this short link into your internet browser to have easier access to links in this book:

https://hudsonandrew.activehosted.com/f/25

Health Check

Before you start this fitness routine - please
consult with your doctor.

- Do not attempt to exercise while unwell.

- Do not carry-on exercising if you feel pain
  - if the pain doesn't calm please tell your
  doctor.

- Avoid exercising after consuming alcohol
  or a large meal within the last couple of
  hours.

- If you take prescribed medication, check
  with your doctor to make sure it is okay to
  exercise.

- If you are in any doubt, go check with a
  doctor. It may be helpful to show the
  doctor the circuit training routines you
  will partake in, if the doctor suggests for
  you not to partake in certain exercises

there are always alternatives that will suit you.

Think before you train. If you are under 16 years old, then I advise you to stay away from lifting weights as your body hasn't fully developed. I 'Andrew Hudson' will not take any responsibility for any physical injuries caused by exercises I have stated in this book – injuries are a part of fitness and can always be avoided so please train responsibly.

Read through the entire book before performing any of the circuits/warmups/cooldowns.

Chapter 1 – Why an Unhealthy Lifestyle is Miserable

Fat is not fun. Most people that are overweight want to lose weight once they realize their way of living is doing themselves some serious harm to them mentally and physically. The reason I say that not all overweight people want to lose weight is because some people are unaware of their lifestyle and some people just enjoy being a massive lump on a massive sofa. If you are reading this book, then I know you are with the majority looking to lose weight. Before you get to the "how to lose weight" part of this book, it is important you know why you need to lose weight and you can use this as motivation for any of the days that you don't feel like getting a workout in or when you're tempted for a quick chocolate bar.

This chapter will lay out why an unhealthy lifestyle is so bad for you and will give you an insight to how your lifestyle will improve once you make changes. I also urge any of you that have friends or family that are overweight but unaware of their weight, to just let them know about their unhealthy ways in a kind manner. Many people don't know that they are damaging their mind and body, just a quick heads up is all it takes is just a quick word to them which will help them out. But if you are unaware of what obesity/ being overweight does to you, you are about to find out...

The Problem of Obesity

The term obese is described as "Grossly fat or overweight", would you be proud of being known as grossly fat?

Everyone falls under these four categories. These categories are underweight, healthy weight, overweight and obese. Your actions in life are what allow you to end up in each of these categories, actions such as eating well and exercising regularly will put you in the healthy weight class and actions like over-eating and exercising once a blue moon will most likely put you in the overweight or obese class.

BMI (Body Mass Index) is how you are measured to be placed in these groups. To calculate your BMI all you need to do is divide your weight in Kg, by your height squared in meters (Weight(kg) / Height^2 (m)). For this book

I want you to use your weight and BMI to track your progress, I think BMI is a great way to track progress as the number is generated from your height and weight, so it is fair to compare with other people at different weights and heights.

If your BMI is between 18.5 and 25 then congratulations, you are considered a healthy weight – a great goal for those looking to get into good shape and also a good goal for those maintaining weight. But please remember just because you are in this weight class, that doesn't mean that you're immune to becoming fat. All it takes in an unhealthy lifestyle to grow out of a healthy weight, so once you reach this BMI, remember to maintain it.

Underweight BMI – If your BMI is below 18.5 then you are underweight. You will want to gain weight, both muscle mass and body fat. If you find yourself in this situation, this book won't help you. Instead, increase your portion sizes and start body weight training.

Overweight BMI – If you have a BMI that is between 25 and 30, unfortunately, you are considered overweight and will need to cut the fat. Luckily, you are currently reading a book that will allow you to cut the pounds so that you get back into the healthy weight section.

Obese BMI – A BMI above 30 means you are obese. Hopefully, if you are in this zone then you will study this book to make a change. There is always time to slim up and lower your BMI, carry on reading and get stuck in!

It's finally time to get into the problems that come with being overweight or obese. These problems are mostly health-related issues, and I cannot say that you are guaranteed to fall victim to them because of your weight, but I can say that the higher your BMI is above 25 then the more likely you will be at a high risk to these fatal health conditions. The health-related problems include:

- Increased chance of cancer.
- High Blood Pressure.
- Increased risk of stroke.
- Increased risk of heart disease.
- Higher chance of Kidney Disease.

I listed the most common and fatal ones but believe me when I say the list doesn't end there. I hope that makes you aware of the danger you are in from your current situation. This should be scary and proves that the benefits of being overweight, which is just being able to be a couch potato, are heavily outweighed by the negatives. If the previous conditions weren't a big enough wake-up call, then I will list a few more mental problems caused by being overweight.

- More likely to be stressed
- Low self-esteem
- Low confidence in certain situations

Yet again just the most common problems listed but that should be enough for you to reconsider your food choices and your lifestyle. If that's not enough to persuade you, there is more to hopefully make you see that your current unhealthy lifestyle isn't working out for you.

The 71.6% of American that are overweight are more likely to need hospital treatment because of their lifestyle, which of course isn't ideal or cheap. This is likely to put you under financial stress, which can be easily avoided from a change to your lifestyle.

Finally, I would like to say how a healthy diet is much cheaper than having all these takeaways and snacks. Although I am going to contradict myself by saying that studies have proved healthy food to be more expensive than unhealthy food. However, it is typical for unhealthy food to be less filling and more addictive which causes the consumer to buy more unhealthy foods. If you look at the prices of takeaways, you can see how quickly they add up to put a dent in your bank balance. A healthy diet contains more filling food which will keep your energy levels high, won't require you to buy too much and will save you money. Later on in this book, the diet section proves how that is the case with examples.

Benefits of Living Healthy

Let me guess, you think that being healthy is awful because of all the general stereotypes that suggest healthy people wake up with a glass of that disgusting green juice and go on a run every day. Well, I want to use this book to prove that's not the case, you can still enjoy the grub every now and then but once you are in the routine of living healthy you will appreciate the switch you made. Here are just some benefits of being healthy that should encourage you to make the switch:

- Feeling more confident.
- Looking slimmer.
- Having more energy.
- Reduces the chance of dementia.
- Reduces the chance of osteoporosis.
- Gives you clear skin.

Doesn't that sound so much better! By exercising and eating well you are expanding your life expectancy and improving the quality of your life. This all doesn't come instantly, you have to give it time and stick to it but I promise you that the results will come.

My Experience of Health & Fitness

I will just give you a brief history of myself, how I was affected by being overweight and how exercise changed my life.

Many years ago, I was fat. My BMI was 26.3 and I always found myself drained of energy after work. Working long days would leave me no choice but to eat junk and train only on the weekends with low energy. I failed countless times at exercising and I would give up midsession, that was because I had insufficient energy levels and couldn't motivate myself to stick to it.

As a simple man, I hated seeing all these weight loss videos on fasting or certain diets, I just wanted a routine I could follow to get myself out of my poor situation. I remember circuit training sessions from school and made many circuits with exercises that I know would make me sweat. After following these workouts and started cutting the junk out of my diet, I got into boxing and found my love for fitness.

As the years have gone by, I no longer struggle with low-confidence levels, being ashamed of my body and being unable to motivate myself. It was thrilling to see how the years of exercise had bettered me as a person, which is why I want to better everyone who reads my books. As a qualified personal trainer and a boxing coach, I enjoy teaching others and I only hope to reach more and more of you out there!

Chapter 2 – What Makes Circuit Training Great for Losing Weight

Introduction to Circuit Training

Circuit training is a workout technique that involves a series of exercises performed in a cycle, with minimal rest in between each exercise. Circuits usually have 4 to 12 exercises in one rotation and can be repeated however many times necessary. Circuit training can be done at home, outside or at a gym. Ideally, you will need a bit of open space. Getting started is always the hardest part and I understand it takes a lot of work to do something that you think you will hate.

Benefits of Circuit Training

Circuit training is honestly fantastic! The pros outweigh the cons by a country mile, I will list a few reasons below that support my statement:

Circuit Training is Practical – Set up circuit training at home, at the gym or outside without worrying. Depending on the equipment required for the circuit it is unlikely to take longer than 3 minutes to get ready and usually takes under 30 minutes to complete. This allows you to fit a training session into your busy schedule.

Circuit Training brings Variety – Circuit training can be set up in any way to train anything. In this book the focus is on weight loss, even though that slightly narrows down what can be trained there are still many exercises that can be used with circuit training. These exercises can be done inside and out, with or without equipment and altered to be time efficient. Here are some ways circuit training can be used for training:

- Improving Aerobic Endurance (Improving Fitness Levels)
- Building Muscular Strength (Gaining Muscle Mass)
- Improving Muscular Endurance (Improving how long muscles can take exercise before getting tired)
- Weight Loss (Burning fat at a steady rate)
- Getting back into a sport after an injury (Recovery)
- Improving anaerobic endurance (HIIT Training, intense fat burning or muscle building)

Circuit Training is for Everyone – That's right, whether the only exercise you do is going to the shop or whether you work out twice a day – circuit training has so many variables that you can change to make it suit you! I would suggest you stop reading this book if you work out twice a day as you will need more of a challenge, my other books may help you!

Circuit Training is Easily Modified – There are many changeable variables that determine how hard you train, how often you train, what you train and so on. Changing the variables is a key part of implementing Progressive Overload. I have listed the variables below:

Circuit Training Variables:
- Number of exercises in the circuit.
- The number of sets.
- The time spent doing each exercise.
- Reps completed for each exercise.
- The time spent resting between each station.
- How long to rest after a set.
- The resistance of the exercises.

- The intensity level you work at during the exercise station.
- What exercises to include.
- How many days a week you train.

Circuit Training is Time-Efficient – Circuits usually last between 20 minutes to an hour, in this book I am to make circuits last roughly 30 minutes as I understand you will struggle with long periods of exercise.

Circuit Training allows you to stay Motivated – There are a few ways to stay motivated using circuit training, other training methods have more limits so that some of these motivation factors wouldn't work. I will now talk about ways to stay motivated.

Motivation

If you are reading this book the chances are that you are overweight, obese or not happy with your shape or size. The first step for change is you reading this book to learn how you can lose weight, the following steps are you exercising regularly, following a diet, staying in routine and this is all possible by staying motivated.

Being motivated is where you have a drive or passion to reach your goal every single day, even on the days or sessions where you've had enough you still push yourself to get it done. Staying motivated is hard, especially if you train by yourself – this is why I am here to offer you tips on how to feel motivated every day until you reach your goals.

Signs of becoming demotivated can be as little as not finishing the last minute of a workout.

Once you start to cut things out of your routine, you will lose weight at a slower rate or start to gain weight if you drop the routine. What I am trying to say is that you must stick to your training and diet plan for a prolonged period, so that you can see the results you are after. Of course, you will not see results after a few days of training, don't let this put you off.

How to Stay Motivated

Motivation is key to continue exercising on a regular basis, it can be hard to force yourself to exercise sometimes but to reach your goals or solve your problems. You have to have the correct mindset in order to continue, without it you will be lost. If you ever feel like not exercising refer to the points below and find that drive deep within yourself.

I believe that getting into a routine is the best way to motivate yourself. Have you heard the phrase '3 weeks makes a habit'? Well once you get into a habit of training you will be in a routine and get used to exercising. It may start off with just 2 days a week which is great as you are building a routine so you can work towards your fitness goals. This is my biggest goal as an author, if I can see people get into a routine then I know a strong foundation is set.

Working out with other people is also a great way to motivate yourself. You won't even realize it but when you work out with a friend or family member you will enjoy it more – a social aspect of fitness is very good as you will be excited to work out again with somebody. You could also have a friendly competition to push each other.

Reward yourself. If you reach your goal treat yourself to something like a night out with friends or family, this may push you to meet your goal. Try not to reward yourself with something that will reverse your progress like a large chocolate cake. Just have fun once your goal is reached.

Make it fun. Many people dread exercising, but if you can find a way to put your own spin on it to make it fun then please go for it as you will enjoy exercising. If you enjoy exercising, then you will have no problem with exercising making you motivated. I have tried to make the circuits involved in this book fun because why would anyone want to do something, they don't find enjoyable.

Example Circuit

Now that the complete basics are covered, here is how I lay out all the circuits involved in this book. I start with listing a few instructions, the first one will be how many sets to complete – this is the number of times you should complete the circuit. Secondly, I state how long to rest in between each exercise, for most circuits it is 30 seconds – please note that this not the same as the rest period between sets.

The rest between sets is longer because you need to recover to get into another circuit, I may also word this as rest for 3 minutes after completing the first set. I then set you a target of what heart rate/training zone you should work at – the previous sub-chapter explains this. I finally state the time it takes to complete the warmup, circuit and cooldown, which all play a part reaching the recommended 150 minutes of moderate physical activity.

Complete 2 sets, rest for 30 seconds between each exercise with a 3-minute rest between each set. Train at the Light Training Zone (Around 60% of Max HR). This circuit takes roughly 20 minutes to complete including the warmup and cooldown.

Warmup 1
1. Pushups – 30 seconds
2. Marching on the spot – 30 seconds
3. Calf Raise – 30 seconds
4. Half Squats – 30 seconds
5. Knees to Chest – 30 seconds
6. Jog on the spot – 30 seconds

Cooldown 1

At the top and bottom of the circuit, I include the phrase "Warmup 1" and "Cooldown 1", to avoid confusion I have that there because it should remind the reader to warm up before the circuit and cooldown after the circuit. "Warmup 1" is the name of a warmup I have provided in this book, you will need to be familiar with the warmups and cool down I provide in this book as you will be doing them before and after every circuit.

Example Six-Week Plan

This is just a short sub-chapter that demonstrates how I lay out my actual Six-week plan in the 7th chapter. Every day is covered, and this should be an inspiration for those who want to create their own six-week plan.

Week 1:

Monday –

What to Train: Train Example Circuit 1

Progressive Overload Changes: No changes to this circuit.

Tuesday – Rest Day

Wednesday –

What to Train: Complete Example Circuit 2

Progressive Overload Changes: No changes to this circuit.

Thursday – Rest Day

Friday –

What to Train: Train Example Circuit 1

Progressive Overload: Instead of resting for 30 seconds, march on the spot. This will keep you working for longer. Please still use the time to rest properly between the sets.

Saturday –

What to Train: Complete Example Circuit 2

Progressive Overload: Make a slight change to this particular circuit by working for 40 seconds on each exercise, this will make you work for longer to complete the circuit and more calories burnt.

Sunday – Rest Day

Week 1 Overview:

On Monday and Wednesday, you will be training the example circuits as normal. On Friday you will modify the circuit so that you spend less time resting by replacing the 30 second rest period by marching on the spot – this light activity still builds up the workload. On Saturday I use progressive overload to the second example circuit by increasing the time spent on exercises to make it harder. You have completed 120 minutes of exercise this week which is getting you closer to the recommended 150 minutes.

After the week's plan, I also include an overview of the week to reinforce the information. I do not provide a certain time for when you train, but I strongly suggest you train between two meals, so you have sufficient energy for before and after the circuit – obviously leave enough time as isn't good to train straight after eating. This is just an example so please don't follow this.

Equipment

Don't worry, this book requires no equipment for completing the circuits. That means you won't have to spend lots of money which is always a bonus. I will list a few things that you may find helpful for when you are working out. You can find links to all the equipment for a reasonable price in the Basic Circuit Training Bundle. Please remember everything below is optional, I want to make exercising cheap as possible so that it gives more people motivation to do so.

- A Smart Watch that tracks your Heart Rate.
- A Stopwatch to help you keep track of how long you exercise for. Can use an app on your phones if it cheaper for you.
- 2kg Hand Weights that you can hold while completing the circuits to make it slightly harder.
- Fitness Matt – Just to make it more comfortable to train on the floor and stops sweat getting on the floor.

- Fitness Attire – Just a pair of shorts and a training top/bra will be suitable for when you are exercising. I link some reasonably priced brands in the basic circuit training bundle.

Chapter 3 – You Are What You Eat

I feel as if this is the part most people are least looking forward to when it comes to making a change to live a healthy lifestyle. But it's not as bad as you may think, you will still be able to taste great food and you will feel an increase in your energy levels. Diet may be hard to stick to, but it really is important and you will learn why. After reading this, you will be aware of what a healthy diet consists of and how it is much different to what you would expect!

The Importance of Diet

If you eat like crap, then you will train like crap – it is as simple as that. Many people underestimate the importance of how you choose to eat and drink. Training will help you get into shape, but if you are going to eat poorly then you may as well not train. A good diet goes hand in hand with training hard.

It can be easy to put on a bit of weight, I do have some sympathy for the larger people as I was once on the heavy side – working full time got me to make poor food choices. I will explain the most common ways of getting to an overweight stage below. The points below also prove a point that you are not overweight because you are unlucky, your choices in life have gotten you to where you are.

Eating poorly – Although this sounds obvious many people don't realize when they are eating poorly. For example, a sugary snack every couple of hours doesn't sound harmful – I can assure you it all adds up to be stored as fat in your body. As you can guess, the more fat stored in your body the rounder you look.

Quick Meals and Snacks – This is a big reason for the millions of overweight people. I used to work a long shift and I know that it is much easier to get microwavable meals and snacks than to prepare nutritional meals. The takeaways and snacks will not provide your body with all the nutrients that are needed, the food is mostly heavily processed, in which you know that is not good for your body.

How much you eat – Even if you eat foods that are considered healthy, it is still possible to get fat by eating too much of those foods. That is why you need to space out when you eat. It will be unrealistic to drastically cut down on how much you eat each day, that why you should eat smaller meals more often every day.

Late-night snacks – Many people think that it is bad to eat anything at night but there is nothing wrong with it. Typically, people make poor food choices later on in the day. You need to remember that calories DO count at night and swap the midnight brownie for a midnight banana.

Lack of exercise – Although this hasn't got much to do with diet, how you eat does affect how you train. A good diet will provide your body with energy so you can train hard. Exercising after eating foods high in saturated fat and sugar will make training very difficult and potentially make you sick – putting you off exercise.

What Your Body Needs

Your daily diet will need to consist of:

- 30% Protein. You can get this from many things like eggs, lean meats, poultry, beans cheese and natural peanut butter.

- 30% Fats. Good fats that contain omega-3 and omega-6 fatty acids are essential for bone, joint, and brain health. Good sources of these fatty acids include fish, nuts, olive oil, flax seeds, or avocados.

- 40% Carbohydrates. Natural carbs like peas, sweet potatoes, beans, nuts, and whole grains.

- 25 grams of Fiber. Fiber helps with digestion and regulating weight. Foods high in fiber are things like fruits, vegetables, whole oats, nuts, and legumes. Many people struggle to consume this much. Fiber is wonderful because it keeps you full up for longer.

- 2.5 liters of water. It is important to stay hydrated, after all, your body is made up of 70% water

Everything that I mentioned above fuels the body's metabolism. It is important that you understand how the metabolism works, in the subchapter underneath I compare the human body to a furnace as it will help you understand the importance of your diet.

How the Metabolism Works

The Furnace Analogy:

The body is just like a fire, it needs fuel to get started. With a fire you need paper, firelighters, sticks, logs and coal to keep it burning. You light the paper to set fire to the firelighters to set fire to the sticks and so on to get to the coal. This will keep the fire lit in the furnace to keep you warm all day. Now let's substitute some things to compare this furnace to your body. Instead of paper you have vitamins, instead of the firelighters you have minerals, instead of sticks we have protein, instead of logs we have carbs and finally instead of coal we have fats. The body needs vitamins, minerals, proteins, carbs and fats to keep the metabolism working hard so that you have enough energy for your body to function to the best of its ability all day long.

The Most Important Meal of the Day

Did your mum tell you that breakfast is the most important meal of the day? Well, your mum is always right after all. A survey showed a couple of years back that 98% of people that live in the UK said they either don't eat breakfast, or they eat what is considered an unhealthy breakfast. Although the percentage may have changed slightly as it's now 2021, this still isn't good enough and links heavily to people generally having no energy all day long.

A healthy balanced breakfast is so important in the morning, think of a healthy breakfast like lighting the fire. The correct breakfast choice will kickstart your day with all the nutrients you need to energize your body – this will allow you to not find yourself tired after waking up and feeling great throughout the day.

Overall, you should take from this that you need to have a healthy breakfast every day and you need to space out meals to keep your energy levels high. If you have low energy all day long you will struggle at work, or to exercise and make things harder for yourself.

Weight Loss Tips

The overall idea of a weight loss diet is to eat a balanced diet and to eat less than your daily recommended calorie intake – for Men: 2500 calories, for Women: 2000 calories. Here are a few tips to consider that will help with weight loss:

- Eat lots of Leafy Green vegetables like kale, spinach, and collards are low in calories and contain a lot of fiber.
- Stay away from eating junk food, allow yourself a cheat day once a fortnight.
- Structure out what you will eat every day, leave 3 hours between each time you eat.
- Try to eat less for each meal but make up for it by having 5 meals a day, 3 of them should be the main meals and 2 of them should be mini meals in between the mains.
- Avoid snacking regularly, snack once or twice a day. Snack on healthy foods like nuts, or protein shakes. Don't tempt yourself with a chocolate bar.

What you should gather from this section is to cut out junk food from your diet, you should ideally have 5 meals a day and have 2 snacks at the most. Fill up your dinner plate with leafy vegetables. Most importantly you should track what you eat every day, track calories by using the app MyFitnessPal on your phone or you can find a calorie tracker spreadsheet in the Basic Circuit Training Bundle.

Eating Before and After Training

Eating before and after training is very important as you will have to fuel your body to perform the exercises and it is recommended to replenish your body with energy and nutrients after a workout. Eat a small nutritional meal roughly an hour before a workout and eat a bigger meal after a workout. A small meal could be like natural Greek yogurt with berries and a larger meal could be like half a chicken breast with pasta in sauce. If you are struggling for motivation, then check out the weeks diet plan.

Diet Plan

For this section, I will include a week's diet plan that you can follow throughout the six-weeks. This is likely to be a big change from your normal diet, instead of me slowly cutting down your snacks and diet I want you to get straight into it and build a healthy habit. Feel free to replace any meals with what suits you – as long as it isn't any junk. This diet plan is suitable for men and women that are planning to lose weight.

Firstly, I would like to start by saying that for every day, you need to consume 2.5 liters of water. This is very important for keeping you hydrated. Secondly, you will need to figure out what your recommended daily calorie intake is. You are all different shapes and sizes which means you need to consume a different number of calories every day to keep your body energized. Please follow this link to discover what your recommended calorie intake is.

https://www.calculator.net/calorie-calculator.html

All you have to do is type in your height and weight, then 4 numbers will pop up, these are recommended calorie intakes. As you are looking to lose weight, I strongly suggest you aim to consume either one of the bottom two figures – either weight loss or extreme weight loss. Now you know how many calories you are aiming to consume every day to lose weight.

This diet plan unfortunately will not be specific to you, unless you happen to require the same number of daily calories as the diet plan provides. I have tried my best to make this a one size fits all diet plan, if the daily calories for this plan exceeds or falls short of your daily recommended calorie intake, please make changes where necessary by increasing or decreasing portion sizes. Please don't feel forced into following this exact plan if you have any allergies or intolerances, there are many alternative healthy meals out there so feel free to make any replacements. This diet plan is just something for you to take inspiration from.

Diet plan: Split up into 5 meals a day with room for one or two snacks. Each day of eating contains roughly 1800 calories. Two cheat meals allowed all week, they are both on Sunday. I also suggest for you to take vitamin and mineral tablets every day. After a while you will get close to reaching your fitness goal, when you get close to the weight you want to achieve you should start to increase your calorie intake slightly, so you don't continue losing weight until you look like a twig.

Monday –

Breakfast (6am-9am): Bowl of Oatmeal with Your Choice of Toppings

Mid-Morning Meal (9am-12pm): Two slices of whole meal buttered toast with a choice of fruit.

Lunch (12pm-3pm): Healthy Lunch Meal

Midafternoon Meal (3pm-6pm): Baked Beans on Toast – Use 2 slices of whole meal bread.

Dinner (6pm-9pm): Healthy Evening Meal

Snacks (Any time): 2 Snacks – Protein Bar & 30 grams of mixed nuts.

Tuesday –

Breakfast (6am-9am): Bowl of Oatmeal with Your Choice of Toppings

Mid-Morning Meal (9am-12pm): Two slices of whole meal buttered toast with a choice of fruit.

Lunch (12pm-3pm): Healthy Lunch Meal

Midafternoon Meal (3pm-6pm): Coriander, Chicken and Rice.

Dinner (6pm-9pm): Healthy Evening Meal

Snacks (Any time): 1 Snack - Protein Shake

Wednesday –

Breakfast (6am-9am): Bowl of Oatmeal with Your Choice of Toppings

Mid-Morning Meal (9am-12pm): Two slices of whole meal buttered toast with a choice of fruit.

Lunch (12pm-3pm): Healthy Lunch Meal.

Midafternoon Meal (3pm-6pm): Chicken Soup.

Dinner (6pm-9pm): Healthy Evening Meal.

Snacks (Any time): 2 Snacks – Protein Bar & Greek yogurt with mixed berries.

Thursday –

Breakfast (6am-9am): Bowl of Oatmeal with Your Choice of Toppings

Mid-Morning Meal (9am-12pm): Two slices of whole meal buttered toast with a choice of fruit.

Lunch (12pm-3pm): Healthy Lunch Meal

Midafternoon Meal (3pm-6pm): Cajan Rice Bake

Dinner (6pm-9pm): Healthy Evening Meal

Snacks (Any time): 1 Snack – Just the Protein Shake.

Friday –

Breakfast (6am-9am): Bowl of Oatmeal with Your Choice of Toppings

Mid-Morning Meal (9am-12pm): Two slices of whole meal buttered toast with a choice of fruit.

Lunch (12pm-3pm): Healthy Lunch Meal

Midafternoon Meal (3pm-6pm): Instant Pot Chicken and Rice

Dinner (6pm-9pm): Healthy Evening Meal

Snacks (Any time): 2 Snacks – 30 grams of mixed nuts x2

Saturday –

Breakfast (6am-9am): Bowl of Oatmeal with Your Choice of Toppings

Mid-Morning Meal (10am-11.30am): Two slices of whole meal buttered toast with a choice of fruit.

Lunch (12pm-2pm): Healthy Lunch Meal

Midafternoon Meal (2.30pm-4:30pm): Chicken and Rice with Broccoli Pesto

Dinner (5.30pm-8:30pm): Healthy Evening Meal

Snacks (Any time): 2 Snacks – Apple Slices with Peanut Butter & 30 grams of Mixed Nuts.

Sunday –

Breakfast (6am-9am): Bowl of Oatmeal with Your Choice of Toppings

Mid-Morning Meal (9am-12pm): Two slices of whole meal buttered toast with a choice of fruit.

Lunch (12pm-3pm): Cheat Meal

Midafternoon Meal (3pm-6pm): Half a chicken breast, chopped and seasoned with 100 grams of basmati rice.

Dinner (6pm-9pm): Cheat Meal.

Snacks (Any time): 1 Snack – Protein Bar.

Diet Plan Overview:

The breakfast is the same every day, but oatmeal gives you that slow releasing energy you need to start your day properly. This will provide you with 200-300 calories, depending on your topping and what milk you mix the oats with. If oatmeal is not your go to meal, you will find a couple of alternatives later on, but most healthy breakfasts have a combination of oats, fruit and a dairy product.

The Mid-Morning Meal is the same meal every day. Two bits of toast buttered with a side of fruit. This is just an energy boost to fill you up until lunch. This meal is around 200-300 calories depending on the fruit – I personally suggest a banana. Treat this meal as a heavy snack, yet again sorry for the lack of variety for your mornings but you can always search up healthy brunch ideas if you are ever feeling bored. This meal would contain 200-300 calories.

Lunch is the meal for the middle of your day, should provide you with plenty of energy and protein. The lunch meals below should fall around 300-400 calories per serving. You can find many examples of what make a healthy lunch meal under the title "Healthy Lunch Meals", so keep reading to find them and fill up your diet plan!

The Mid-afternoon meal is just another light meal to keep you going until dinner, this usually contains a light chicken dish with a side of rice/veg/pasta but remember you can make adjustments if you don't like what is described on the diet plan. This meal offers roughly 200-400 calories and will keep your energy levels high.

Dinner is the final meal of the day and should be the biggest. As you can probably see by looking at the diet plan, it just states Healthy Evening Meal. You will find a large variety of evening meals that can fill in that spot in the diet plan, pick out some of the meals that you think look good. This meal should contain roughly 400 calories with a high amount of protein.

Snacks are also optional; I would certainly have no more than 2 a day and keep them healthy. You can find snacking options later on in this chapter for inspiration, the snacks will range from 200 to 400 calories. Snack whenever you feel like you need an energy boost, I would suggest that you snack after dinner or snack around your workout if you are exercising that day – I will state more information on when to train in the six-week plan for each day. I also suggest splitting up your snacks – by this I mean that you don't have both snacks in one sitting.

Healthy Meal Alternatives

Most days in the Diet plan repeat "Healthy Lunch Meal" and "Healthy Evening Meal". This doesn't really mean anything when reading it the first time, but you will find all the meals that fit under this category. The reason I structured this chapter like this is so that you have plenty of alternatives for each meal without getting confused. If you are reading from the Print Copy, I suggest for you to download the free eBook that comes with this so you can easily access all the links. Alternatively, you can go to the references to type in the link or search each individual meal listed.

Breakfast alternatives:

Granola with yogurt and berries

Healthy cereal that includes Muesli, Bran flakes, cornflakes. (Roughly 190 calories per serving with milk)

Healthy Lunch Meals:

Tomato Quinoa Soup

Charred Shrimp and Avocado Salad

Grilled Steak Tortilla Salad

Tapas Salad

Butternut Squash and White Bean Soup

Grilled Chicken Sliders

Summer Minestrone

Roasted Salmon with Green Beans and Tomatoes

Crispy Tofu Bowl

Summer Pesto Pasta

Very basic quick meals (What I tend to eat almost every day):

Chicken and rice – Half a chicken breast chopped and seasoned with 100g of basmati rice.

Sausage and Pasta in tomato sauce – Two sausages with around 100g of pasta in a tomato sauce that I get from the shop. Very basic but also tasty.

The recipes for the meals I have included are below:

Baked Beans on Toast – Very simple. Heat beans in a saucepan, toast whole meal bread then butter the toast and put it all together.

Coriander Chicken and Rice

Instant Pot Chicken and Rice

Cajan Rice Bake

Chicken Soup – I think the tins of chicken soup from the supermarkets are easy and affordable to prepare and eat.

Chicken and Rice with Broccoli Pesto

Half a chicken breast chopped and seasoned with 100 grams of basmati rice – This is my personal favorite, I use "chicken seasoning" that can be found in supermarkets and it takes 10 mins to prepare.

I want to include the most options for dinner as eating the same thing each week can get boring. In the plan I list "Healthy Evening Meal" – this is very broad and doesn't exactly tell you what to eat. That's why I am going to list many meals below that fall under that category, you can simply just prepare and eat the meals that I list below. I will also link a recipe with the meal, I am not exactly a cook myself so I will not list difficult recipes. Calories for dinner range between 200-500 calories. (The recipes are from UK websites so keep that in mind for the measurements)

Healthy Evening Meals:

Vegetable Burritos

Healthy Chicken Casserole (390 Calories)

Courgette Pasta Bake

Weight Watcher Cajun chicken recipe

Chili con Carne

Spring Chicken Soup

Ground Turkey Bolognese

Cheesesteak stuffed peppers

Skinny Alfredo

Honey Walnut Shrimp

Thai Style Chicken Salad

Cauliflower Mac n' Cheese

Crispy Chicken with Roasted Carrots and Couscous

California Chicken Flatbread with Chipotle Ranch

Honey Garlic Salmon

Cheat Meal – Can be anything you please because you deserve it. I allow two cheat meals a week, I believe that is fair and won't reverse your weight loss progress. Calories unknown – that's for you to record. Although this is a cheat meal, don't go over the top by eating triple what you would usually eat in a day because you would most likely throw that back up!

Keep in mind the serving sizes of the recipes above. You can substitute other ingredients if you feel like it works. I thought I would provide these links to offer you variety, but you can be like me and live off chicken, rice and vegetables. I like to add leafy green vegetables to all my meals, so maybe you can as well. Now you have so many options which should end your takeaway habits.

Healthy Snacking Options:
- Protein Bar (140 calories)
- Protein Drink Mix (108 calories)
- 30g Mixed Nuts (Around 200 calories)

- Apple Slices with peanut butter (200 calories) – 1 medium apple with 15g of natural peanut butter.
- Greek Yogurt with Mixed Berries (150 calories) – 100g of natural Greek yogurt and 50g of berries.

Chapter 4 – What to do Before and After Exercise

Before you get into the circuits, you must know how you can prepare for them. It is not advisable to get straight into a circuit, going straight into an workout (circuit) is risky because you are more prone to injury. It is just as important to look after yourself after a workout by completing a cooldown. I will list 2 easy warmups and 1 cooldown that you can use before and after each circuit.

Warmups

Before each workout, it is important that you complete a warmup. The idea of a warmup is to loosen up the muscles and slowly raise your heart rate to get you ready for exercise. A typical warmup should include heart raisers and stretches which usually lasts 3 to 5 minutes. I will list a couple of different warmups below that you can complete before a weight loss circuit. I have included how to complete all the warmup exercises in Chapter 8.

Warmup 1 (3 Minutes) – Should be very light.
- Walking on the spot – 30 seconds
- Arm Swings – 30 seconds
- Overhead Triceps Stretch – 15 seconds each arm
- Child's Pose – 30 seconds
- Standing Hamstring Stretch – 15 seconds each leg

This warmup will need to be completed before the Very Low Impact Circuits 1 and 2.

Warmup 2 (4 Minutes) – Should be a light warmup.
- Marching on Spot – 1 minute

- Arm Circles – 30 seconds
- Left Right Floor Taps - 1 minute
- Quad Stretch – 15 seconds each leg
- Cross Body Shoulder Stretch – 15 seconds each arm
- Chest Expansion – 30 seconds

You should be completing this warmup before the Low Impact circuits and the Medium Impact Circuit.

Cooldowns

Cooldowns take place after the workout and typically last 3-5 minutes. Cooldowns allow gradual recovery of heart rate and blood pressure. Cooldowns help you relax after a workout so that your recovery time will improve. Cooldown exercises range from light activity to seated stretches. I will list a simple cooldown below. Remember to check chapter 8 for the exercise descriptions. This should be completed after every circuit.

Cooldown 1 (3 Minutes) – Aim to lower your heart rate slowly.

- Light March on Spot – 30 seconds
- Close the Gates – 30 seconds
- Shoulder Shrugs – 30 seconds
- Shake off the body – 30 seconds
- Seated Spinal Twists – 30 seconds
- Seated Hamstring Stretch – 15 seconds each leg

Rest and Recovery

Tips to help with recovery:

- Replenish Fluids. During a workout, your body will use up lots of fluid for energy. You ideally need to refill during exercise but if you replenish after you will get a great recovery boost. Replenishing fluids is like drinking water or healthy supplements such as protein shakes.

- Resting and relaxing - You need to allow your body time to recover after a workout, this is because your muscles are likely to be slightly damaged after a workout – if you continue to train on the slightly damaged muscle then you will make the damage worse and put yourself at risk of an injury. Hopefully, you know how to rest and relax – may just be like sitting around at home.

- Cooldown – Just covered this but a good cooldown will lower the chance of injury and keep the muscles in good condition.

- Ice bath – May sound unpleasant but the coldness will make the muscles feel less sore.

- Water therapy – This is where you have a shower with hot water for 2 minutes and cold water for 30 seconds, repeat 4 times. The reason for that is that the difference in temperate will repeatedly constrict and dilate blood vessels to flush out waste products in the tissues.

- Sleep – Aim for 8 hours every night, your body produces growth hormones while you sleep which is mainly responsible for growth and repair.
- Avoid Overtraining – You want to train hard but not too hard, it will take your muscles longer to recover if they are extremely worn. You will also risk injury which may take you weeks to recover from.

If you are injured, then recovery is very important. Use the tips above to speed up your recovery time so you can get back into training quicker. Younger people and athletes are more likely to have a better recovery time, anyone can still improve their recovery time by training more often and using the tips. Do not try to exercise too soon after an injury or a workout as you will not have recovered and will be likely just to get an injury, be patient and slowly get back into it until you feel confident you are ready to train hard again.

As you exercise throughout your life your recovery time will progressively get better. I will suggest a few supplements that will help you with quicker recovery but it isn't exactly needed at your level. Protein is the nutrient that helps rebuild muscle so fill up on protein shakes and meat!

Summary

Overall, exercising is more than just working out a few times a week. You will have to change the way you live essential by eating healthier and preparing for workouts by warming up and cooling down. I guarantee if you follow this you will reduce the risk of getting injured, this is a big positive as you will be able to continue circuit training and feel great about yourself for doing so.

Chapter 5 – The Training Basics You Need to Know

This chapter will focus on helping you make progress towards your fitness goals. In this chapter, you will discover how the intensity of your workouts can be calculated, how the intensity will help you make progress, how training zones work, why progressive overload is the driving factor to making progress with weight loss and finally how to avoid injury.

Intensity

Intensity is simply a variable in circuit training that is a measurement of how hard you are working. Intensity is a variable that can be measured by heart rate. The harder you work while exercising the higher your heart rate will be. It is known that the fitter the individual is the harder it is for them to raise their heart rate, that's why if you are overweight it will be relatively easy for you to raise your heart rate.

The ways you can work harder by exercising depends on how you are exercising. If you are running then run faster, if you are weightlifting then lift heavier and so on. For circuit training, the best way to work harder is to decrease the time spent resting between exercising and you can also try to fit in more reps in the 30 seconds of exercise or you could add an extra exercise to your circuit. There are so many ways to make it harder and that's why I love circuit training.

Training Zones

There are 5 training zones, each training zone determines how hard you are working while exercising. This uses your active heart rate to put you in a zone. Before training, athletes will set a goal of what training zone they will want to stay in during their workout,

Very Light – 50-60% of max heart rate. This is for when you slowly raise your heart rate during a warmup or for people recovering from injury. Walking is an exercise in this range.

Light – 60-70% of max heart rate. This is also known as the fat-burning zone. You should be able to exercise at this level for long time, this zone will help you burn fat and improve muscular endurance. A good warmup would take place in this zone.

Moderate – 70-80% of max heart rate. This zone is great form improving blood circulation around your heart and skeletal muscles, you will get a bit of a sweat on from this zone. Training in this zone is also good for burning fat.

Hard – 80-90% of max heart rate. You will breathe harder and work aerobically. At this intensity, you will improve your speed endurance and get used to having lactic acid in your blood. I do not recommend working in his zone for a long period as this may result in injury.

Maximum – 90-100% of max heart rate. Your body will be working at maximum capacity, you can only train in this zone for short periods of time as lactic acid builds up quickly in the blood and can cause cramp or injury. Working in this zone is unsustainable.

For this book, I suggest that you never work harder than the moderate zone (Over 80% of max HR). Start by working in the light zone and remember to use warmups to slowly raise your heart rate to the correct zone. When you look at the circuits it will state which training zone to exercise at.

How to Calculate Heart Rate

You will need to be able to track your heart rate during exercise for you to stay on track in the same training zone. The best way to measure your heart rate is to buy a smartwatch that can measure your heart rate, it may be slightly pricey but once you have it, life will be easy as you can track your heart rate while exercising- the smartwatch may also include many other benefits that will help you with your fat burning journey. You don't have to pay for a smartwatch, you can measure by counting your pulse in a minute after the workout, but this is long and tedious.

You may be wondering why you should only work in a particular training zone, well this is because working outside of your training zone will make it too hard or too easy for you. If you find the training is too easy then you will not make any gain towards your goal of losing weight, because you will not be using as much energy your body will store that unused energy as glycogen and if too much glycogen is stored then it is stored as fat for the long term. If you end up storing more fat then you obviously won't be losing much weight. Training should be hard but not so hard that it is unbearable, if you find yourself almost breathless, on the verge of vomiting or a certain body part hurts then stop as you will just cause your body harm. This links to injury which I cover further on.

In order to work in the training zone that suits you then you will need to know your max heart rate. You can work this out with a simple math equation, 220 – (Your Age) = Your max heart rate. It is as simple as that, your max heart rate is the number of times that your heart can beat in a minute while your body is working at maximum exertion – working at max exertion is something that I strongly suggest for you not to try, only extreme athletes will work at this level as they have the training and experience.

You will use your max heart rate to work out what heart rate you should be working between. I will use the light training zone as an example here. So, I am 26 years old meaning that my max heart rate is 194bpm (220-26=194). To find the lower percentage of the training zone (60% for the light zone) you will have to do divide your max heart rate by 100 and times that new number by 60 (194 / 100 = 1.94 X 60 = 116.4 bpm), next you will do the same but times that number by 70 instead of 60 (194 / 100 = 1.94 X 70 = 135.8bpm). This means for me to work in between the light zone I will have to keep my heart rate between 116 bpm and 136bpm. I hope you understand how to use this to calculate other training zones.

Progressive Overload

Progressive overload is when the workload for a training session increases over time as the athlete adapts to training. Progressive overload is mainly used for strength training but can be used for helping with weight loss as well. If you decide to complete the same circuit 3 times a week for 6 weeks then yes you will get fitter, however you will not be able to get as fit as you could potentially be. For example, if an experienced athlete and a complete beginner both went into a room and completed 30 jumping jacks under the same conditions then the beginner will have a higher heart rate than the athlete as the athlete's body has adapted to exercise over all the years of training – therefore the athlete would have to work harder to get to the same heart rate as the beginner.

That should give you the idea that if you become fitter while training the same circuit then you will have to make it harder, if you just continue to train the exact same circuit then you will notice that your heart rate will gradually get lower each week while training. Progressive overload is the action of making the workouts harder each week so that you maintain the heart rate you need to work at. Working at the same heart rate will increase the rate of you losing weight. Below will be a short example of how you can implement progressive overload in circuits over time.

Week 1 - (Train Example Circuit 1) – Rest for 30 seconds between each exercise, complete 2 sets with a 3-minute rest between each set. Train at 60% of Max HR.

Warmup
1. Jumping Jacks – 30 seconds
2. Pushup – 30 seconds
3. Sit-ups – 30 seconds
4. Heel Flicks on Spot – 30 seconds

Cooldown

Week 2 - (Train Modified Example Circuit 1) – Rest for 30 seconds between exercises, complete 2 sets with a 3-minute rest between each set. Train at 60% of Max HR.

Warmup
1. Jumping Jacks – 45 seconds
2. Pushups – 45 seconds
3. Sit-ups – 45 seconds
4. Heel Flicks on Spot – 45 seconds

Cooldown

The six-week plan does not look like that as writing out the circuit for every day you are training would double the length of the book and I would rather get all the information over to you in the shortest book possible. But as you can see for the second week the exercises are 45 seconds long, this makes it harder than the first circuit as the exercises are only 30 seconds. Remember that is just an example just to show you how it works, in the six-week plan the progressive overload instructions are clear and easy to follow.

Injury Prevention

Injuries must be avoided at all costs. There are many injuries that you can get from training – the most common injuries for beginners are muscle strains. As your coach I want you to avoid all injuries at all costs. Injury can be very painful and may require hospital time if serious – I don't want you to experience pain and certainly have to spend time in hospital which may cost money for people in other countries. Injury is also a setback, you cannot train while injured for obvious reasons – this will stop your routine of training and losing weight.

Ways to Prevent Injury:

- Have the correct diet – Look at the diet section of this book for a refresh on what you should be eating and drinking. Your muscles need the energy to contract repeatedly during excrcise. Consuming too much food every day would increase your chance of vomiting as the excess food isn't being used as energy it is just sat in the stomach weighing you down, not eating enough will put your body into a catabolic state meaning that your body will be unable to properly repair tissue damage.

- Warming up before exercise. If you go straight into a hard workout then your muscles will be tight and more likely to strain if overstretched during exercise.

- Cooling Down after exercise – you need to allow your body to recover slowly.

- Have rest days – As a beginner, you should certainly not try to exercise every day as your body will not be used to it and you will be likely to pick up an injury. If you are getting started only exercise 3 or 4 times a week.

- Don't Train Through Pain – If you encounter pain while exercising then you are likely to have picked up an injury, do not continue to train as you will make the injury worse.

- Improve Flexibility – If your muscles have an extended range of motion that means it will be harder for them to get strained or pulled – the usual result of an injury. Stretching consistently will improve your flexibility, my circuits will also improve flexibility.

- Don't Train if Unwell – You will need to give your body time to recover from an illness as your body will constantly be working hard to fight away the illness. You may have low levels of energy when unwell making it difficult to train anyway.

If you feel like you have slight pain or injury just check with your doctor if you will be able to carry out the circuits provide. Now that I have covered all the important information, this is where the fun starts. The next chapter contains the circuits.

Chapter 6 – The 5 Starter Circuits to Accelerate Weight Loss

Here is the part you have all been waiting for, this is the chapter that contains 5 circuits that can be done at home with no equipment. All you will need is a bit of open space and maybe a fitness mat to stop the floor from getting sweaty, don't exercise around furniture or valuable items just in case something gets broken, or you trip over.

I assume that you are overweight, and you have little experience when it comes to exercising. That is not a problem as that will change. I will have 2 very low impact circuits, 2 low impact circuits and a medium impact circuit that you can follow depending on your level. As a personal trainer, I am used to having the client right in front of me so I can coach them based on the ability they can show me, in this instance I cannot see what ability you are at. That's why this book has lots of variety within the exercises and intensity. Every exercise will be explained with a photo to show the demonstration in chapter 8.

You can mix and match the exercises from different circuits to make it suit you, as long as you follow a fitness routine then you are taking a step in the right direction to lose weight. The circuits will work out the entire body so that the weight loss will be much more noticeable. Work at the best level for you and do your best!

Stretches
Just before you get into the circuits, I am aware that as beginners you are more likely to have problems that restrict you from exercising to the best of your ability. The most common are joint issues which won't allow you to complete

floor or low exercises with comfort, I want to offer common stretches and exercises that you can perform every day to strengthen your weak points so that you are ready to exercise. This isn't an alternative to the warmups, this is for those who struggle with the circuits.

Below is a list of stretches, each stretch will show which part of the body it targets and how it helps strengthens the joints. Hold these stretches for as long as you can, each day you stretch you should hopefully feel stronger in certain joints and more flexible.

Lunges – This stretch will strengthen your knees. These lunges will be slightly different from lunges that are included as an exercise in circuits throughout the circuits, these lunges are slower so that the quadriceps, hamstrings, calves, glutes are all strengthened which will make your knees and ankles stronger. To do a stretching lunge start by standing with legs shoulder-width apart, then take a big step with your left foot forwards and bend your knees into it, you will feel the stretch and hold this stretch for 10-15 seconds before stepping back and swapping legs. Place a hand on the floor to help you balance if needed, the photos below should help you find the form.

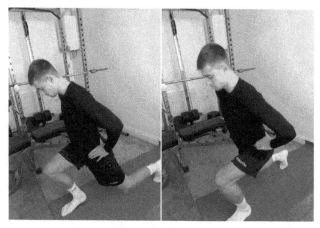

Hip Swings – This will allow you to have extended motion in your hips which prevents stiffness and pain. How to complete: Stand in an open space next to a wall, chair or something that can support your balance. Make sure that the open space is in front and behind you because you need to slowly swing your left leg forwards and back for around 30 seconds while keeping your other foot planted on the floor, remember to switch legs afterward and do the same for 30 seconds with the other leg.

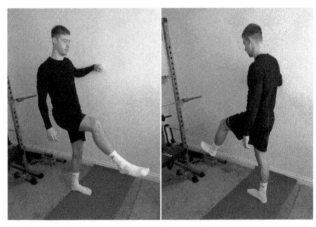

Quadricep Stretch – The benefits of stretching quads are that it helps you maintain balance, keeps your legs strong and decreases the chance of injury. You can discover how to stretch your quads in chapter 8 under the warmup exercise descriptions. The only difference is that you should hold the stretch for longer if you are trying to build up strength.

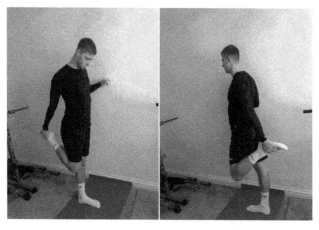

Shoulder Rolls – Improves range of mobility in shoulders. How to do it: Stand straight with arms straight down your side, then roll then forwards 10 times and backward ten times like the photo shows below. You can use your arms to create momentum to make the shoulder roll. The photo is hard to show how to do it, but hopefully you get the hang of it.

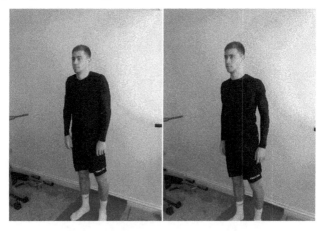

Try to complete these stretches every day so that you can build up the strength that will prepare you for the beginner circuits. If you are getting started and you feel like it is necessary for you to stretch every day for a couple of weeks before getting into the circuits then do it – you can use the two weeks to also fully focus on sorting out a healthy diet to follow in which you will hopefully be stuck to a healthy routine by the time you start training.

I suggest you spend 10 minutes a day on stretching, so split those stretches up whatever way suits you the most. Try not to push yourself too hard, these stretches should only be light. These stretches do not appear in the six-week plan, although lunges are involved in a circuit.

Very Low Impact Circuit 1

I recommend this to everyone as it is a good starting point to see where you are at. All the exercises in this circuit will be standing exercises, if you have joint problems then definitely stick to this circuit until you build up enough strength to move on. Remember, you and your doctor know your own body better than I do.

Complete circuit twice. Rest for 30 seconds in between each exercise and rest for 2 minutes after completing the first circuit. Train at Light Training Zone (Around 60% of Max HR). This circuit will last roughly 25 minutes including warmup and cooldown.

Warmup 1

1. Marching on the spot – 30 seconds
2. Half Lunges – 30 seconds
3. Hand Raises – 30 seconds
4. Side-to-side steps – 30 seconds
5. Hamstrings and rows – 30 seconds
6. Arm Circles – 30 seconds
7. Half Squat – 30 seconds
8. Knee Repeaters Left – 30 Seconds
9. Knee Repeaters Right – 30 seconds

Cooldown 1

Very Low Impact Circuit 2

The same difficulty as the first Very Low Impact Circuit, the difference being that some of the exercises are different to provide that variety. This also contains no floor exercises where you would need to bend low to complete meaning this will be easier to complete for those with joint problems.

Complete two sets. Rest for 30 seconds between each exercise. Rest for 2 minutes after completing the circuit then go again for the final set. Train at the light Training Zone (Around 60% of Max HR). This circuit will take roughly 30 minutes to complete including the warmup and cooldown.

Warmup 1

1. Marching on the Spot – 30 seconds
2. Shoulder Raise Half Lunge – 30 seconds

3. Open Gates – 30 seconds

4. High Knee and Backwards Kick – 30 seconds

5. Straight Punches – 30 seconds

6. Body Twists – 30 seconds

7. Box Step – 30 seconds

8. Knees to Hands – 30 seconds

9. Side Lunges – 30 seconds

Cooldown 1

Low Impact Circuit 1

Now you are looking at the step up from very low impact circuits, these exercises require more muscle groups to work and they will be worked harder than previously.

Repeat the circuit twice. Rest for 30 seconds between each exercise and rest for 2 minutes after completing the first set then go again. Train at light training zone (Around 65% of

Max HR). This circuit will take roughly 25 minutes to complete including the warmup and cooldown.

Warmup 2
1. Bounce on the spot – 30 seconds
2. Knees to Chest – 30 seconds
3. Jumping Jacks – 30 seconds
4. Sidestep Squats – 30 seconds
5. Uppercuts – 30 seconds
6. Knee Pushups – 30 seconds
7. Up and Out – 30 seconds
8. Left Right Floor Tap – 30 seconds

Cooldown 1

Low Impact Circuit 2

Repeat circuit 3 times. Rest for 30 seconds between each exercise and rest for 2 minutes between sets. Train at the light training zone (Roughly 65% of Max Heart Rate). This circuit will take just under 30 minutes to complete including the warmup and cooldown.

Warmup 2
1. Open the Gates – 30 seconds
2. Stage 2 Pushups – 30 Seconds
3. Ankle Taps – 30 Seconds
4. Double Sidesteps – 30 seconds
5. Plank – 30 seconds
6. Twist and Punch – 1 minute

Cooldown 1

Medium Impact Circuit

This is the hardest circuit in this book, if you are looking for harder circuits move on to the next book in this series. Not to worry as this circuit can still be done by beginners and can also be modified to suit you. There are two harder circuits in the Basic Circuit Training Bundle.

Complete 3 sets, rest for 30 seconds between each exercise. Rest for 2 minutes after each set. Train at the moderate training zone (Around 70% of Max HR). This circuit will take roughly 30 minutes to complete including the warmup and cooldown.

Warmup 2

1. Jogging on the Spot – 30 seconds
2. Russian Twists – 30 seconds
3. Lunges with twists – 30 seconds
4. Straight Punches – 30 seconds
5. Lying Superman Hold – 30 seconds
6. Tuck Jumps – 30 seconds
7. Crunches – 30 seconds
8. Squats – 30 seconds

Cooldown 1

How often to train

Before I waffle on, the next chapter contains a six-week plan which will sort out your diet and training routine for the next 6 weeks. Now that's out the way, I can show you how often you can train these circuits if you decide not to follow the six-week plan.

If you are a complete beginner then you will want to train 3 times a week with the very low impact circuits, gradually over a few weeks you will want to be able to complete 4 circuits a week. Start by training Monday, Wednesday, Friday. You will not need to train more than 4 times a week until you reach a level where you are comfortable to do so, you are the only person who knows when they are ready to make things harder. Ideally, I want everyone to work towards training for 30 minutes five times a week – this will meet the weekly recommended requirement of 150 minutes plus you will certainly be in good shape. I am not expecting you to get to that stage after a few weeks, that's why my follow up books will help you achieve this goal.

Chapter 7 – The 6 Week Workout Routine

I have seen many people transform their bodies in six weeks and you are about to do the same thing. You will now go through the six-week plan, it is easy to follow and can will allow you to progress your fitness levels. The plan is clear to show where progressive overload has been used, what days to train and not train, with an overview of each week which will remind you to track progress. You are not to stop training after the six-weeks, this is to get you started in a routine and you can carry on towards your goals afterward by purchasing the next book or continuing with your own version.

First of all, I ask you to start this routine on a Monday, no better way to start the week. From this Monday you will **not** break your new diet and you **will** stick to your training routine. It's your job now to put in the work and watch it pay off. If you don't feel you are ready for this six-week plan, then remember to stretch every day and try to complete a very low impact circuit a few times before getting into this. Build yourself up to it.

Six-Week Training Plan (Week 1 – The Start)

Please train on the days it tells you to because it allows time for rest and recovery. For when you train on the day is completely up to you – I suggest you pick a time between two meals so you will have sufficient energy for it. I usually train after dinner and I make sure I have a snack for after the workout. That applies for all the weeks! Also, double-check which circuit to train as I have realized it is very easy to mix up "Very Low Impact Circuit 1" and "Low Impact Circuit 1".

Monday –

What to Train: Complete the Very Low Impact Circuit 1 as normal. (Complete to the best of your ability)

Progressive Overload Changes: None as it is just the first week.

Tuesday – Rest Day. Remember to try some of the recovery tips I listed earlier, this will prepare you for tomorrow's session.

Wednesday –

What to Train: Complete Very Low Impact Circuit 2 as normal

Progressive Overload Changes: This circuit is slightly harder but no changes to the actual circuits.

Thursday – Rest Day

Friday -

What to Train: Complete Very Low Impact Circuit 1.

Progressive Overload Changes: No changes. Try to see if you can complete more reps of certain exercises in the 30 second periods.

Saturday – Rest Day.

Sunday – Rest Day. Great work for this week, now it's time to get onto week 2.

Week 1 overview:

You shouldn't have found this extremely difficult, but if you did don't worry - all I suggest you repeat this week until you feel comfortable with going on the next week. You would have completed 85+ minutes of moderate exercise. Will increase this over time so you work towards the recommended 150 minutes of activity. No progressive overload changes yet.

Week 2

Monday –

What to Train: Complete Very Low Impact Circuit 2.

Progressive Overload Changes: Just like last Friday, try to complete more reps in the 30-second exercise period but this is just a suggestion.

Tuesday – Rest Day

Wednesday –

What to Train: Complete Low Impact Circuit 1

Progressive Overload Changes: As this is a harder circuit please complete this to the best of your ability with no changes.

Thursday – Rest Day

Friday –

What to Train: Complete Very Low Impact Circuit 1

Progressive Overload Changes: This is easier than low impact circuits, so this time spend 40 seconds on each exercise and keep every other variable the same. This will slightly increase the time you spend exercise making you burn more fat.

Saturday – Rest Day

Sunday – Rest Day. Cracking Stuff. Hope you are working well and most importantly getting it done at your own pace – onto week 3!

Week 2 Overview:

This week should be a slight step up from the first week. I include a new circuit into the plan "Low Impact Circuit 1", this is a slightly harder circuit than the very low impact circuits. I also increase the exercise period in the very low impact circuit 1 to make it harder. You would have completed 90+ minutes of exercise this week.

Week 3

Monday –

What to Train: Complete Low Impact Circuit 2

Progressive Overload Changes: None to this circuit, train this as normal.

Tuesday – Rest Day

Wednesday –

What to Train: Complete Very Low Impact Circuit 2

Progressive Overload Changes: Again, spend 40 seconds on each exercise with 30 seconds rest to increase the time that your heart is pumping quickly for.

Thursday – Rest Day

Friday –

What to Train: Complete Low Impact Circuit 1

Progressive Overload Changes: No new Changes to this circuit.

Saturday –

What to Train: Complete Low Impact Circuit 2

Progressive Overload Changes: No changes to the circuit, but you should notice an extra day of training for this week and the weeks to come.

Sunday – Rest Day. But today I urge you to try water therapy from the Rest and Recovery section because of the extra training load.

Week 3 Overview:

This week is a bigger step up with the difficulty to implement progressive overload, this is because you will be training 4 times a week from now on. This adds up to roughly 115+ minutes of moderate exercise every week, well on the way to meeting the recommended 150 minutes of recommended exercise each week. I also introduce Low Impact Circuit 2 this week, get used to it!

Week 4

Monday –

What to Train: Complete Very Low Impact Circuit 1

Progressive Overload Changes: Lower the resting time from 30 seconds between each exercise to 20 seconds, make sure you allow proper rest in this period as it now starts to get tough.

Tuesday – Rest Day

Wednesday –

What to Train: Complete Low Impact Circuit 1
Progressive Overload Changes: Spend 40 seconds on each exercise, just like how you do for the very-low impact circuits.

Thursday – Rest Day

Friday –

What to Train: Very Low Impact Circuit 2
Progressive Overload Changes: Lower the resting time from 30 seconds between each exercise to 20 seconds.

Saturday –

What to Train: Low Impact Circuit 2

Progressive Overload Changes: Increase the time spent on each exercise by 10 seconds, meaning you exercise for 40, rest for 30.

Sunday – Rest Day

Week 4 Overview:

This week I made the circuits harder to complete by reducing the rest time on the very low impact circuits and for the low impact circuits, I increased the exercise periods. The weekly exercise duration will be a few minutes less than last week as I reduced the rest period – so around 110+ minutes of exercise for the week.

Week 5

Monday –

What to Train: Low Impact Circuit 1

Progressive Overload Changes: No new changes from last week – keep it up!

Tuesday – Rest Day

Wednesday –

What to Train: Low Impact Circuit 2

Progressive Overload Changes: No new changes from last week. Still exercise for 40 seconds each time.

Thursday – Rest Day

Friday –

What to Train: Low Impact Circuit 1

Progressive Overload Changes: Complete Circuit in moderate training zone (Around 70% of max heart rate). This requires you to work harder during each exercise, you can do this by completing more reps of the certain exercise in the same 40 second period.

Saturday – Rest Day

What to Train: Low Impact Circuit 2

Progressive Overload Changes: Complete at 70% of Max HR like the other Low Impact Circuit.

Sunday – Rest Day

Week 5 Overview:

For this week, I have stopped putting the very low impact circuits in the plan as I feel that these won't provide a real challenge to you unless modified to a large extent. However, I did modify the Low Impact Circuits by asking you to complete the circuits at 70% of your Max HR. You will get a sweat on for 110+ minutes this week.

Week 6 – Final Week

Monday –

What to Train: Low Impact Circuit 1

Progressive Overload Changes: Continue to work in the moderate training zone, the new addition will be that you should lower the rest period from 30 seconds to 20 seconds. The rest period between sets will stay the same.

Tuesday – Rest Day

Wednesday –

What to Train: Low Impact Circuit 2

Progressive Overload Changes: Continue to work in the moderate training zone, just reduce the resting duration to 20 seconds like the other low impact circuit.

Thursday – Rest Day

Friday –

What to Train: Medium-Impact Circuit

Progressive Overload Changes: Complete this circuit normally, this is a reasonably difficult circuit so do your best.

Saturday –

What to Train: Low Impact Circuit 1

Progressive Overload: No new changes, train this exactly like you trained on Monday. See this as a slight recovery session.

Sunday – Rest Day. The last day of the six-week plan but not your last day of training.

Week 6 Overview:

Firstly, I want to congratulate you on getting this far. It is a real achievement to try something new and stick to it. I hope that you notice positive changes with your body and you are in a great training routine now of exercising 4 times a week. So well done, I am proud of you. Remember to contact me or the Facebook group for additional help.

This is the only week where I introduce the medium impact circuit, this is a harder circuit so that is one of the ways I have implemented progressive overload. Another way I increased the difficulty was by increasing the length of the exercise period – this also means you exercise roughly 115+ minutes a week.

Although this is the final week, this doesn't mean that you stop after this week. You can continue to train by looking at how I have made the plan and how I made it harder. Or you can crack onto my second book of the series that will pick it up from this moment. How you train is up to you, as long as you stick to it and see the results then I have no problem. I suggest working your way towards training 5 times a week or getting to 150 minutes of moderate exercise each week.

Chapter 8 – How to Complete Every Exercise for the Circuits

No messing around, I will list each exercise and explain it in this chapter. Some may have photo examples to help you get the correct form. The form is very important because if you do not complete reps for certain exercises correctly then it is likely you will pick up an injury. Check out @dec.beales on Instagram, I would like to thank him for demonstrating all of the exercises for me.

For the majority of the exercises, I start by describing the starting position, the picture for that is below. That is what I mean by standing straight with feet shoulder-width apart. This will not apply to the floor exercises.

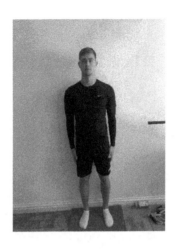

Very Low Impact Exercises

    Marching on the spot – Stand straight with feet shoulder-width apart. Start on your left leg by raising your left knee and right arm. Raise your leg to a point where you feel comfortable, then, lower your right arm and left leg so you can repeat on the alternative side. The photos below should help, marching should be done in a smooth motion. This exercise is light but gets you moving and your heart pumping.

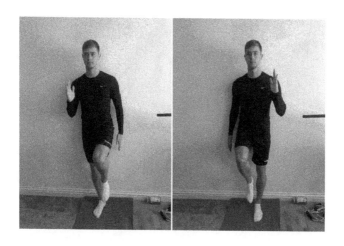

Half Lunges – This is the easier version of lunges. Stand straight to start, step out with your left foot and place it down, facing forwards. Keep your right foot planted then slightly bend both knees and place your weight onto your front leg. Hold that position for a second or two before stepping back with your left foot and repeating with your right leg. Alternate sides for 30 seconds. This exercise strengthens your legs (Quads and Calves) and will get the blood pumping around your body.

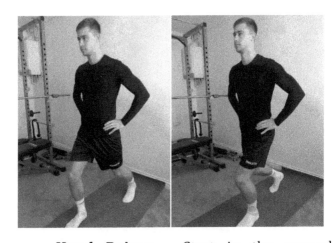

Hand Raises – Start in the normal standing position and hold your hands out to the side like shown in the left picture. Then raise your hands as high as possible (shown in the right picture), once in that position, lower your hands back to the starting position and continue to raise and lower your hands. Continue to repeat this for 30 seconds and feel free to march on the spot at the same time if you find this too easy.

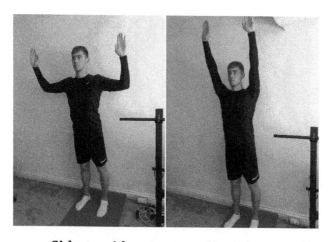

Side-to-side steps – Start by standing straight with feet apart. Firstly take a step to the right with your right foot and slightly bend your knees into it(the 3rd picture shows this), from the right step position step to the left with your right foot and place your foot next to your left foot(2nd picture), then step left with your left foot and bend your knees into it like the 1st photo shows. Once you get into the rhythm it will become natural and is a real fun cardiovascular exercise. Repeat this for 30 seconds by going from right to left, then left to right and so on...

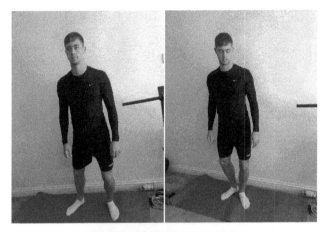

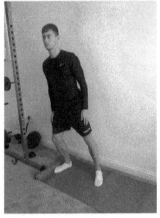

Hamstring and Rows - The pictures should help you with this. Stand straight, keep arms down in front of you - pretend that you are holding onto a pole with your hands. Pull up as if you are rowing a boat, at the same time kick your left leg back so your heel is flicked towards your bum. Then lower your left foot to the floor while pushing down with your hands back to the starting position and repeat with your right foot. Continue this left-right-left movement for 30 seconds. This is a fun exercise to strengthen your legs and get you sweating.

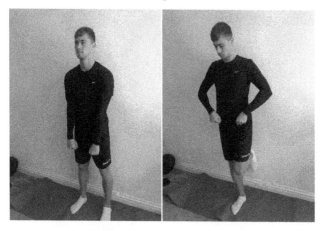

Arm Circles – Start by standing tall and bring your arms out straight on either side so that you are shaped like a capital "T". Imagine that you are drawing circles with your fingers, start by drawing small circles then slowly make your circles bigger. You will be using your shoulders to get the circular motion in your arms, switch direction after 15 seconds. You can choose how small or big you draw your circles as long as you keep them rotating. The pictures below should help, from isn't all too important as long as you are rolling your shoulders to reduce stiffness in your upper body.

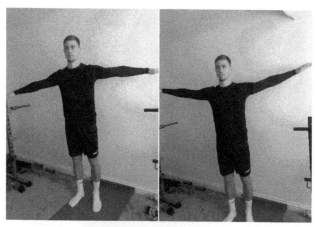

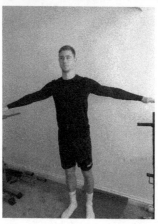

Half Squat - Start with feet shoulder-width apart and slightly turned outwards. Put weight into your heels, sit your bum back and bend your knees slightly until you get to a position which the 2nd picture shows, afterwards push up with your legs to stand back in the starting position. Don't bend knees too much for this level as you may find it painful when getting back up. You can put your arms out in front of you like the photos shows for balance support. You should keep squatting down and pushing up for 30 seconds, will increase muscle mass in your legs as it works your calves, hamstrings, glutes and quads.

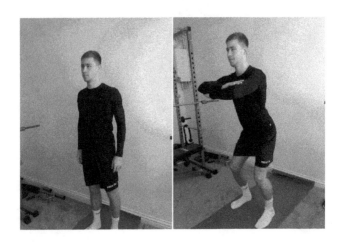

Knee Repeaters Left - Start by standing in a half lunge position in which your left foot is placed much further back than your right foot. Keep both legs slightly bent and hold your hands out in front like the 1st photo shows below. Then bring your left knee to your hands and after they connect place your foot back in the starting position. Your right foot should stay planted while you continuously move your left knee forwards and back for 30 seconds. This exercise is great for improving your balance, flexibility in your hips and mainly strengthens your core. Apologies about the angles of the photos, they both work the same leg.

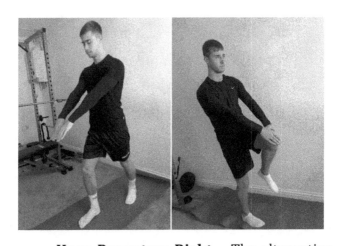

Knee Repeaters Right – The alternative to Knee Repeaters Left. Start by standing in a half lunge position but have your right foot placed much further back than your left foot. Then bring your right knee to where you hold your hands out in front, once they connect place your right foot back in the starting position. Remember to keep your left foot planted and repeat for 30 seconds. This has the same benefits as "knee repeaters left". Both exercises should be included in the same circuit if you are making your own to provide balance. Sorry about the angle again.

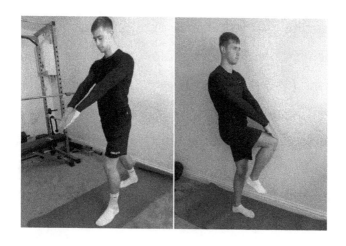

Very Low Impact Circuit 2 Exercises

Shoulder Raise Half Lunge – This is a combination of hand raises and half lunges. Start in the usual standing position, with hands up by your side like you're surrendering (2nd photo). Of course, you're not going to surrender because you should step backward with your left foot and at the same time raise both your arms up either side of you as far up as possible (3rd photo). Hold for a second before stepping your left foot back into the starting position and lowering your arms. Then step back with your right foot while raising your arms (1st photo), finally step forwards into the starting position and lower arms. Repeat this for 30 seconds, remember to swap legs each time. This exercise will improve your overall coordination and will work major muscles in arms and legs.

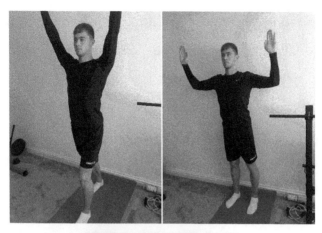

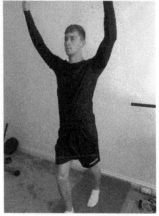

Open Gates - Start in the casual starting position. Lead with your left leg, imagine you are drawing the letter 'n' to your left. Do that by raising your left knee in front of you then twist your hip to rotate your leg 90 degrees to the left and then lower your leg. Repeat this on the right side. The photos below will help your form, switch legs every time you open the gate and repeat for the time given. Will reduce stiffness in your hips/groin and improve balance.

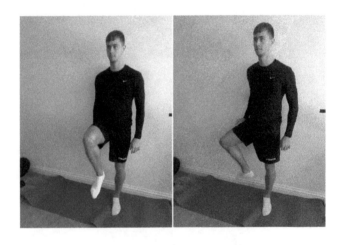

Straight Punches – Start by standing in a causal boxing stance, do this by placing your weak foot (pointing forwards) in front of your strong foot (facing outwards) with your arms held high and fists clenched like the 1st photo shows below

– always keep your knees slightly bent. To throw a left straight punch then simply extend your left arm out quickly until you cannot extend your arm anymore, which then you should instantly bring your arm back to the starting position – always keep a clenched fist and the punch should be like a snap. To throw a right straight punch, follow the same steps as the left straight punch but twist your body while the punch is thrown. My boxing book can always help you with form. The benefits from this include faster hands, will make you sweat and potentially hand eye coordination. Repeat left-right-left-right straight punches for the time period.

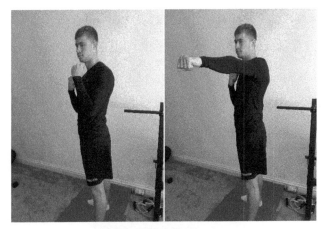

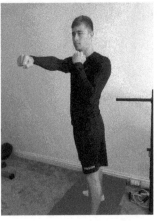

Body Twists – Start by standing with knees slightly bent and feet shoulder-width apart. Hold your hands together in front of your torso. Keep your feet planted on the ground, then use your arms and lower back to twist your body slowly from side to side. Repeat that motion for the time given. This exercise is great for strengthening your abs/core, lower back and improving flexibility.

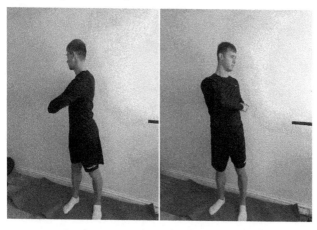

Box Steps – Stand with feet slightly wider than shoulder-width apart. Then from that position step forwards with your left foot while keeping your knees slightly bent (1st photo), then step forwards with your right foot so you are in a sort of half squat position (photo 2), then step back with your left foot followed by your right foot to get back to the starting position. Practice the steps slowly until you get into rhythm, once you get the hang of it exercise in the circuits for the time given. This exercise is good for strengthening leg muscles.

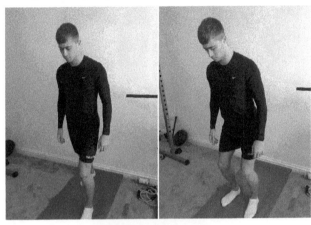

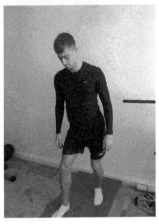

Knees to hands – Stand straight with feet slightly wider than shoulder-width apart. Hold both hands out straight in front of you as shown below. Then raise your left knee to your right hand and lower it back to starting position after touching. After you have lowered your left leg, raise your right knee to your left hand then lower your right leg after they connect. Will be like a crisscross. Carry this exercise out for time given, great for burning belly fat, improving balance and strengthening obliques.

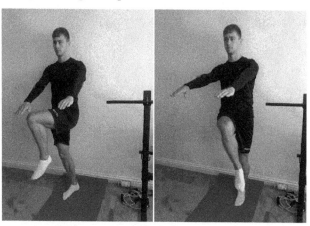

Side Lunges- Begin by standing light on your feet with feet slightly apart. Lunge left by stepping as far as you can left with your left foot and bend your left knee into it. Keep your right leg straight, your feet should always face outwards and always face forwards. From that position keep your feet planted to the ground, lean to the right side and switch your legs so that your left leg is now straight and your right leg is bent. Continue to switch from side to side, this exercise will work your core, quads and glutes. The pictures below should help.

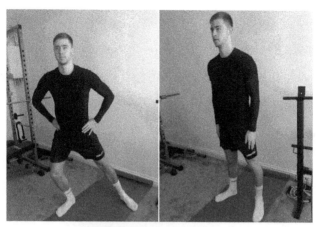

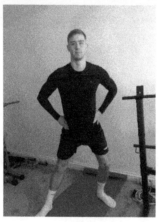

Low Impact Exercises

Bouncing on the spot – Very simple. Stand normally with feet shoulder-width apart and stand on your tiptoes. Then press up and down repeatedly with your tiptoes so that you are bouncing slightly. Try not to let your heels touch the floor. No photo provided due to the simplicity of it.

Knees to chest (Floor) – Lay on the floor facing the ceiling. In one motion: Bring your knees up towards your chest using your hips and core, then hold onto your legs like the 2nd photo shows for a couple of seconds before letting go and returning to the laying-down position. Continue that movement for the time allocated for exercise. Make sure you use your core to get your knees up and this exercise is brilliant for improving flexibility and core strength.

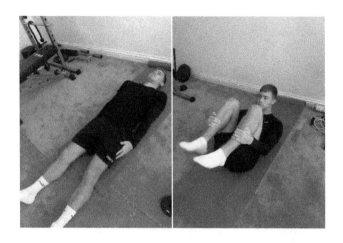

Jumping Jacks – Start standing with feet together and arms down by your sides (Photo 1). In one motion bend your knees and spring up into the air, separate your legs and raise your hands so your body is in a star shape. Land in the star shape (Photo 2) and from this position spring up again to get yourself back into the starting position by lowering your arms and closing legs. Repeat this motion, this exercise is very good for cardio which contributes towards burning calories and fat.

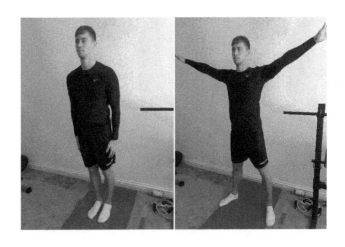

Sidestep Squats – Very similar to side to side steps. Start as normal and carry out the side to side steps. Every time you step to either side you need to slightly squat on the transition of stepping to the side, for example, if you are about to step to the left you will want to slightly bend your knees before you place your left foot on the ground. The pictures should help. This will work the main leg muscles, core and lower back. Sidestep squat from left to right, then right to left on repeat until done.

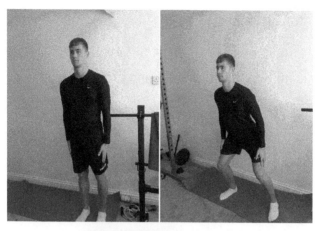

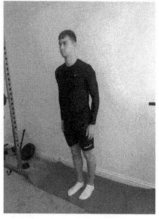

Uppercuts – Get into the causal boxer stance that I previously explained with the "Straight Punches" however you can keep your guard lower. Punch up in the air with both arms in the order of left-right-left-right, you will need to lower your arm after every punch so you can punch again. The form is not that important for this instance, but you will get a sweat on. Try not to punch too high, if you are looking to into a mirror then your punches should stop around your chin.

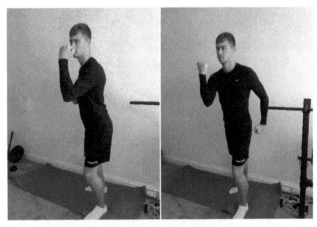

Knee Pushups- Place both knees on the floor and your hands on the floor so that your body is kept off the floor. From this position lower your chest to the ground by bending your elbows, once your chest is close to the ground use your arms to push up back to the starting position. Continue to lower and raise your chest using your arms for the time given, having your knees on the ground makes this exercise easier because you will have less of your body weight to push up. Will strengthen your triceps, pectorals and shoulders as well as maintaining your higher heart rate.

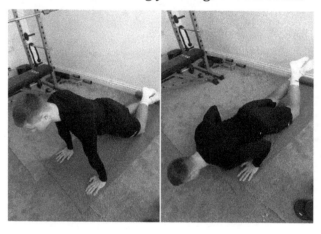

Up and Out – Start in the usual standing position. Start on the left side by stepping to the left while extending your arm to the left and point your finger like the 1st photo shows, from that position bring your left foot forwards and bring your left hand to the sky (2nd photo). Keep your right foot planted in the same position for the entire time. Repeat these steps alternatively for the right side, it may look like you're dancing in the sixties. Just a fun cardiovascular exercise.

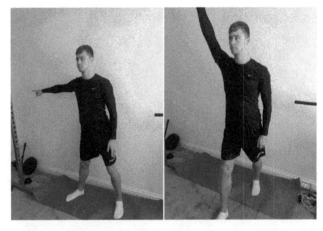

Left Right Floor Tap – Begin by standing with legs slightly bent and your hands down by your sides. Reach down with your left hand and tap the floor to the left of your left foot, stand back up and repeat this but tap with your right hand to the right side of your right foot. Continue this motion for the time given. Remember to bend your legs when bending down to avoid back injuries. Strengthens lower back.

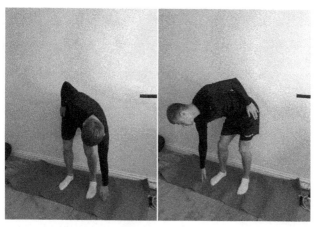

Low Impact Circuit 2

Open the gates – Previously Explained, description found under the "Very Low Impact Exercises".

Ankle Taps – Begin by laying down on the floor facing the sky. Keep your arms by your sides as you need to mainly use your arms in this exercise. Your feet should be planted on the floor. To complete an ankle tap: Reach for your left ankle with your left hand and try to tape your ankle, remember to stay in the initial laying position. Afterwards, bring your left hand back while reaching out to tap to your right ankle with your right hand. This exercise is great for strengthening obliques. Continue to tap both ankles for the time given.

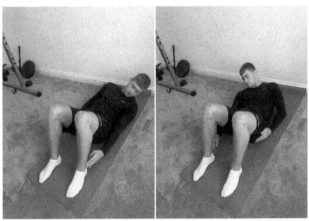

Double Sidestep- (Make sure you have plenty of space) This is just a sidestep which is previously explained, the difference being you are required to sidestep in each direction twice before switching direction. For example, from the starting standing position you will step left with your left foot, bring your right foot across and then step left again before switching direction. This is a fun cardio exercise which will improve your agility. No photos provided as it would look just like a normal sidestep.

Plank- Begin by laying on the floor facing the floor and keep your forearms flat on the ground underneath your chest along with the rest of your body. To get into the plank push up slightly with your forearms and your feet so that the only parts of your body connecting with the floor are your arms and tiptoes. Hold this position for the time given if you can, feel free to go onto your knees if you find this too difficult. This exercise is fantastic for our entire body, but most importantly burns belly fat and builds up abs. The photo below shows the plank in action, don't raise your bum too high while planking as that is cheating, you should feel the burn.

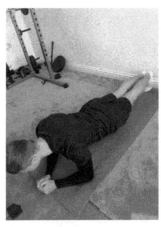

Twist and Punch – Begin in the position that picture 1 shows, to do this place your left foot in front of your right and point it forwards, extend your arm out in front of you with your fist clenched and your right foot should be back at a 90 degrees angle to the right so that you're stood side on. To get to the stance of picture 2, step back with your left foot so that its pointing to the left while bringing your fist back to your chest, then step forwards with your right foot and extend your right arm like you are punching. Continue to switch stances for the time given, will improve coordination and get you sweating.

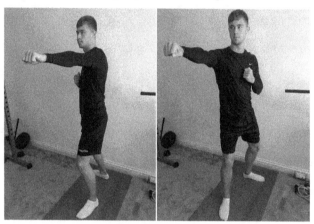

Medium Impact Exercises

Jogging on the Spot – Light run on the spot, just transfer weight from one leg to the other repeatedly. No picture included, c'mon everyone knows how to jog on the spot.

Russian Twists - Start in a sitting position so that your body and upper legs are in a "V" shape, to do this sit up on the floor while slightly leaning back, have your knees slightly raised and bent (1st photo). Start on the left side by holding your hands together next to your left hip, use your core and lower back to twist your body from left to right and use your hands to tap the floor either side of your body. Tap from left to right, right to left for the time given. Cross your ankles if you feel it help you balance. This exercise strengthens obliques, abs and lower back.

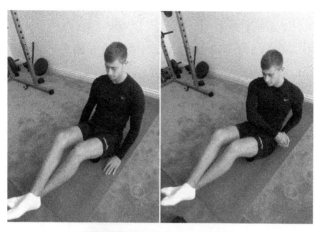

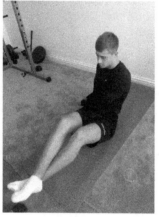

Lunges with twists- The lunge has already been described as a stretch in this book, however there are 2 differences. The first difference is that you will not hold the lunge for as long as you would if you were stretching.

Secondly, every time you lunge forwards, your will use your lower back and arms to twist your body left then right before standing back up in the starting position. This exercise is almost an entire body workout that improve balance, flexibility and strengthens your lower body.

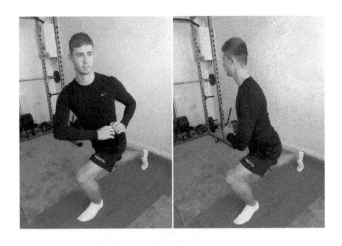

Straight Punches – This has been previously explained as a very low impact exercise, the only difference is that you will be throwing the punches slightly faster to keep your heart rate at the moderate training zone.

Lying Superman Hold – Starting position: Picture 1 shows that you should lay down facing the floor with your arms slightly in front of you bent and your legs slightly apart while relaxed. Then use your core and back to raise your arms and legs off the ground, hold this position for a second or two before relaxing your muscles back into the starting position. Continue this for 30 seconds, a great core exercise.

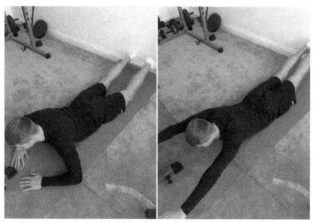

Tuck Jumps – From the usual standing position bend your knees slightly and push through your heels to jump up into the air, once your feet have left the ground tuck your knees into your chest by bending them. Be careful as you need to prepare for the impact of your fall so don't spend too long in the tuck position. This exercise will build up power in your leg muscles, along with help you burn fat and allow you to get worn out quickly. Don't worry about trying to jump as high as dec here!

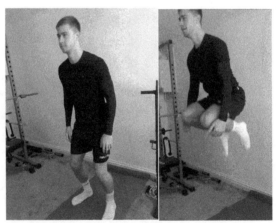

Crunches – Start by laying on the floor facing the sky with your arms crossed over your chest. Bring your knees up and make sure your feet are together while planted on the floor. From this starting position use your core and lower back to bring your chest about halfway to your knees, once you reach this point slowly release and lower yourself back to the ground. Complete as many as you can in the time, this will let you build up abs and burn belly fat.

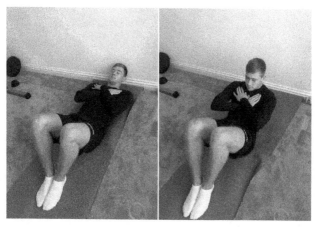

Squats –Start with feet shoulder-width apart and pointing outwards. Put weight into your heels, sit your bum back and bend your knees to lower yourself until your thighs are almost parallel to the floor, from this position push up through your heels to complete a squat. Keep your arms out in front of you while doing this to improve balance and avoid this exercise if you have knee problems. This exercise is brilliant for building stronger legs.

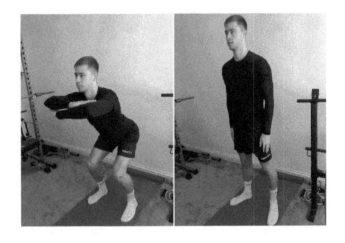

I have now described every exercise used in this book. More Exercises and Descriptions are available in my other books or the Basic Circuit

Training Bundle. More descriptions are below for the Warmup and Cooldown exercises.

Warmup Exercise Descriptions

Walking on the spot – Self-explanatory. Pretend you're walking slowly by lifting and lowering your left leg then right reg, feel free to actually walk around if you have space for it.

Arm Swings – Start with arms by your side and simply swing both arms up as high as you can and back down again. Keep swinging for 30 seconds.

Overhead Triceps Stretch – To stretch left arm: Lift left arm up straight and bend your elbow, reach as far down your back as you can with your left hand. Then push down on your left elbow with your right hand to stretch your triceps. Hold for 10 – 15 seconds then repeat with your right arm by completing the steps alternatively.

Childs Pose – This is great for your back. Get into a kneeling position and place hands on the floor in front of you. Then stretch your arms forwards by shuffling your hands across the floor. You will feel your lower back being stretched, hold this for as long as you can in 30 second period.

Standing Hamstring Stretch – To stretch left leg: Start by standing up straight, then bend your right knee slightly while extending your left leg so your left heel is on the floor and your toes are pointing upwards. Hold this stretch for 10-15 seconds then switch leg by repeating steps alternatively. If you don't feel anything the press your hands above your knee on your bent leg as this force will certainly stretch the hamstrings.

Marching on the spot – Already described at the start of this chapter. March for 60 seconds.

Arm circles – Previously explained as an exercise, this time just move your arms slower in circles than normal.

Left Right Floor Taps – Find the description earlier on in this chapter. Complete at a very light intensity for 60 seconds.

Quad Stretch – This requires a good level of balance so try to get something sturdy to lean on. Start standing in the usual position. Bring your left heel to your bum and hold it there with your left hand, use your right hand to lean on a sturdy object and hold this for 10-15 seconds. Swap to your right leg afterward. Pictures for this are found under "Stretches" in chapter 6.

Cross-body Shoulder Stretch – Can be done standing or sitting. Start with your left shoulder: Bring your extended left arm across your torso so your left hand is past your right shoulder. With your right wrist, you want to press on your left wrist towards you so that you feel the burn in your left shoulder. Repeat this but follow the steps alternatively to stretch your right shoulder. Hold this for 10-15 seconds each arm.

Chest Expansion – Dynamic Stretch. Start by standing straight with your arms extended in front of you together like you have just clapped. Keep arms extended, separate your arms and bring them back as far as you can until your chest is puffed out. Hold that position for a second before bringing your arms forwards and your hands together. This should be done all in one motion, keep repeating for 30 seconds.

Cooldown Exercise Descriptions

Light March on Spot – Just a slower version of marching on the spot, which I have already described.

Close the Gates – Start by standing in the usual position. Start with your left leg: Twist your body 90 degrees to the left and lift your left knee upwards, then rotate your hips to bring your knee parallel to your other knee and then bring your foot down. Switch legs and complete the steps but alternatively, do this for 30 seconds and if it helps it is the opposite movement to opening the gates. (A previously described exercise/stretch)

Shoulder shrugs – Can be done standing or sitting. Simple keep your arms down by the side of you and shrug your shoulders up and relax to bring them down. You can also roll your shoulders back to get an extra range of motion. Very similar to shoulder rolls, the only difference being is that you don't have to push your shoulders back to bring them down.

Shake off the body – Just get the blood flowing around the body by shaking your arms and legs. Do this how you like, there isn't really a correct form for it.

Seated Spinal Twists – Sit on the floor with a straight back. Simply just twist your body using your lower back to the left then right repeatedly but slowly. Use your arms to help twist your body. Do this for 30 seconds. This will improve flexibility in your lower back.

Seated Hamstring Stretch – Sit on the floor with back straight and legs extended. Reach forward with both hands and try to touch your toes while keeping legs straight, no worries if you can't touch your toes but just reach as far forwards as you can and hold it for 10 seconds and repeat that twice in the 30 second period.

Chapter 9 – What's Next for Your Future of Fitness?

As you know, this book has a target audience for people who hardly exercise – it is hard for me to know the exact shape and size of the readers, but I will assume you are heavier than the average person. There is no problem with that as this particular book will slim you down to get out of the blob shape to a healthier shape.

After the six-week plan, I hope that you have made progress with weight loss so you can carry on to the next book – a next book you may ask?

"Intermediate Circuit Training", this is the sequel to this book that you are reading now. This next book will be able to take your training further by increasing the difficulty of the workouts, the strictness of the diets and more tips to help you get into the shape you want. I believe this book to also be very beneficially for readers mentally, reading the parts about mindset will hopefully change your outlook on your unhealthy lifestyle.

The final book of this series will be for getting into insane shape. I used HIIT styled circuits that will definitely get you into a defined shape. But you will have a long way to go from here.

Obviously, you don't have to buy my books. You can simply just continue to train how you are at the moment – whether you use my help or not is up to you. I just hope that my message has got across to you – Please stay in a training routine because once you fall out of a routine it is much harder to get back into one. Remember, some exercise is better than no exercise and 2 cheat meals is better than 7 cheat meals a week.

Your Free Gift

The gift you'll receive is an eBook titled: The Circuit Training Weight Loss Bundle. This eBook contains many extras to help you lose weight at a quicker rate and be on top of your progress. In the beginner section of this book, you'll discover:

2 Extra Circuits that you can complete at home, these circuits are slightly more advanced than the ones provided in this book to encourage progression.

Secondly, you will find a checklist full of the optional equipment included in this book. Each piece of equipment has a link to where you can buy it a reasonable price. A list of all the optional equipment all linked. This will allow you to find the equipment for a reasonable price.

You will also find a food budget tracker - a spreadsheet that will allow you to keep track of how much you spend on food with the goal to help you save money in a healthy fashion.

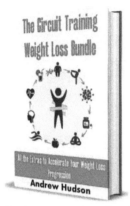

Follow this link to receive the free eBook:
https://hudsonandrew.activehosted.com/f/33

Join the Workout for Weight Loss Community

Living a healthy lifestyle is difficult, especially when you feel as if you are doing it all alone. That's why I suggest for you to join a community of others who are in your situation, this community "Workout for Weight Loss" will provide you with daily posts about weight loss and there will be many people that you can talk to, share experiences with and receive help from.

I aim to post twice a day, providing you with tips, tricks, motivation, workouts, diet plans and so much more to help you lose weight. Not to mention that I may host a few book giveaways every now and then. In a community, your chance of reaching your goals is much stronger and you may make many new friends in the process!

So, if you are looking for that extra help, please join my Free Facebook Group: https://www.facebook.com/groups/workoutforweightloss

Conclusion

Thank you for making it to the end of Circuit Training for beginners! I hope that you enjoyed this book, and you can take the information to help you reach your fitness goals. Remember that losing weight is not a race, it's more of a marathon, so please take it at your own pace and stick to it. I would suggest your next step would be to carry on reading this series and getting straight into the second book "Intermediate Circuit Training".

This book covered the complete basics of exercising using circuit training. I started this book laying down some hard-hitting stats and facts about obesity and why the people who find themselves in an overweight/obese state should make a change. In the second chapter, I list the basics of circuit training including the variables, the benefits, an example circuit, an example week plan and the short list of equipment that can help you while training. In the third chapter, I talk about how important diet is when it comes to losing weight and helping you with training. Also, in this chapter I provide a week's diet plan that you can choose to follow. The diet plan is very broad because there are many people different shapes and sizes with different intolerances and what not so it would be very hard to make it specific while suiting everyone Chapter 4 is the chapter where I talk about how things outside of training like warmups, cooldowns, resting and recovering contribute to you getting the best results possible. Chapter 5 focuses on injury prevention, how to implement progressive overload and the training zones so you can work efficiently towards your goals.

Chapter 6 is where the fun starts as I list 5 circuits at different difficulties that you can do at home with no equipment – train how you like and you have the choice whether to participate in the six-week plan. There are many basic stretches in this chapter as well which can help you build up strength. That links nicely to chapter 7 where I have the six-week training plan laid out. Chapter 8 contains all the exercise descriptions, most of them including pictures which the amazing Dec Beales modelled. Chapter 9 is a short chapter that informs you to not stop and gives you the option to take your training further. That was a brief overview of the book to refresh your memories.

As a personal trainer, I find it much easier to train people 1 to 1 as I can see how they train and the progress they make. However, although writing allows me to reach more people, I sadly cannot see who I am training so that's why I cannot aim this book for people at a certain weight and whatnot. I hope that I have helped in some way and if you read this and feel like it doesn't work for you then no worries – at least you gave it a go.

My other two books on circuit training may also be helpful for you so please give them a read, it would mean everything. It is now up to you to push yourselves further and I support you in every step of the way.

Finally, if you found this book useful in any way then an honest review on this would be greatly appreciated. Feedback is greatly appreciated as it allows me to pass on information in the most effective way to help people reach their goals.

My Books

The Chump to Champ Collection

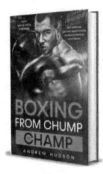 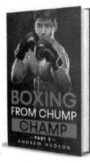 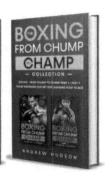

The Weight Loss Circuit Series

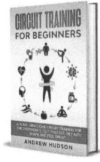 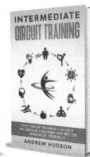 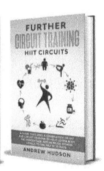

References

Dec Beales - Model for the Exercise Demonstrations.

https://www.instagram.com/dec.beales/

Your Free Gift – The Circuit Training Weight Loss Bundle.

https://hudsonandrew.activehosted.com/f/33

Join the Facebook Community.

https://www.facebook.com/groups/workoutf orweightloss

Follow my Facebook Page.

https://www.facebook.com/andrewhudsonbo oks1

Email me for extra support.

andrew@hudsonandrew.com

BMI calculator. (n.d.). Patient.Info.

https://patient.info/doctor/bmi-calculator-

calculator

Recommended calorie intake. (n.d.). Calculator.Net.

https://www.calculator.net/calorie-

calculator.html

Obesity problems. (2019). NHS.

https://www.nhs.uk/conditions/obesity/#:~:t

ext=Being%20obese%20can%20also%20inc

rease,coronary%20heart%20disease%20and

%20strok

Procon.org. (2016). *Global obesity population*.

Obesity.procon.

https://obesity.procon.org/global-obesity-

levels/

M.L. (2019). *Training recovery*. Verywellfit.

https://www.verywellfit.com/ways-to-speed-

recovery-after-exercise-3120085

J. (2017). *Healthy lifestyle benefits*. Themarlowclub.

https://themarlowclub.co.uk/top-ten-

benefits-to-keeping-fit-and-healthy/

Why circuit training? (n.d.). Miamiathleticclub.

https://www.miamiathleticclub.org/stories-

news/fitness/why-circuit-training-5-reasons-

to-use-it-in-your-

workouts#:~:text=Circuit%20training%20is
%20a%20high,for%20variety%20in%20you
r%20workouts.

D.B. (2020). *Progressive overload*. Healthline.

https://www.healthline.com/health/progressi

ve-overload

Injury prevention. (2017). Healthychildren.

https://www.healthychildren.org/English/hea

lth-issues/injuries-emergencies/sports-

injuries/Pages/Sports-Injuries-

Treatment.aspx

Bodyproject. (n.d.). *Some circuit exercises (video)*.

Youtube.

https://www.youtube.com/c/BodyProjectcha
llenge

A. (2020a). *Floor exercises*. Stylesatlife.

https://stylesatlife.com/articles/floor-
exercises/

A.G. (2021). *Lunch ideas*. Goodhousekeeping.

https://www.goodhousekeeping.com/food-
recipes/healthy/g960/healthy-lunch-ideas/

M.L.C. (2020c). *Chicken + rice meals*. Delish.

https://www.delish.com/cooking/g177/chick
en-rice-recipes/

M.F. (2020c). *Healthy dinner ideas*. Delish.

https://www.delish.com/cooking/recipe-
ideas/g3733/healthy-dinner-recipes/

M.A. (2021b). *More healthy dinner ideas.*

Countryliving.

https://www.countryliving.com/food-

drinks/g4288/healthy-dinner-recipes/

F.S. (2019a). *Healthy snacks.* Healthline.

https://www.healthline.com/nutrition/29-

healthy-snacks-for-weight-

loss#TOC_TITLE_HDR_5

Lightning Source UK Ltd.
Milton Keynes UK
UKHW011828020522
402378UK00002B/358